The Funny Side Collection

The Fart Side

Blowing in the Wind!

(Expanded Full Blast Edition!)

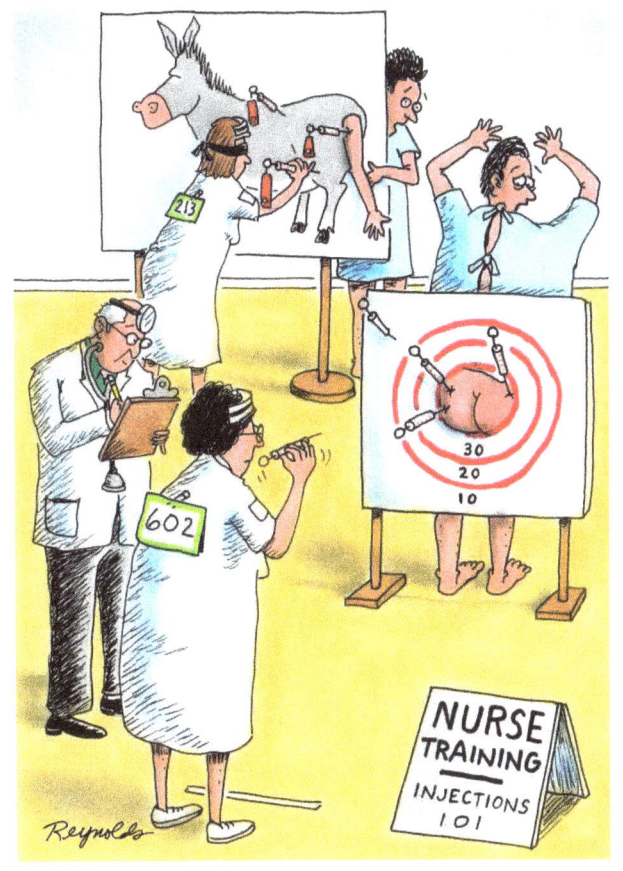

Dan Reynolds
Joseph Weiss, MD

© 2017 Dan Reynolds
       Joseph Weiss, M.D.
       SmartAsk Books
       Rancho Santa Fe, California, USA
       www.smartaskbooks.com

All rights reserved. No part of this book may be reproduced, reused, republished, or retransmitted in any form, or stored in a database or retrieval system, without written permission of the publisher.

ISBN-13: 978-1-943760-58-9 (Color Print Expanded)
ISBN-13: 978-1-943760-63-3 (e-Book Expanded)
ISBN-13: 978-1-943760-13-8 (Color Print Pocket Rocket)
ISBN-13: 978-1-943760-36-7 (e-Book Pocket Rocket)

The Fart Side: Blowing in the Wind!

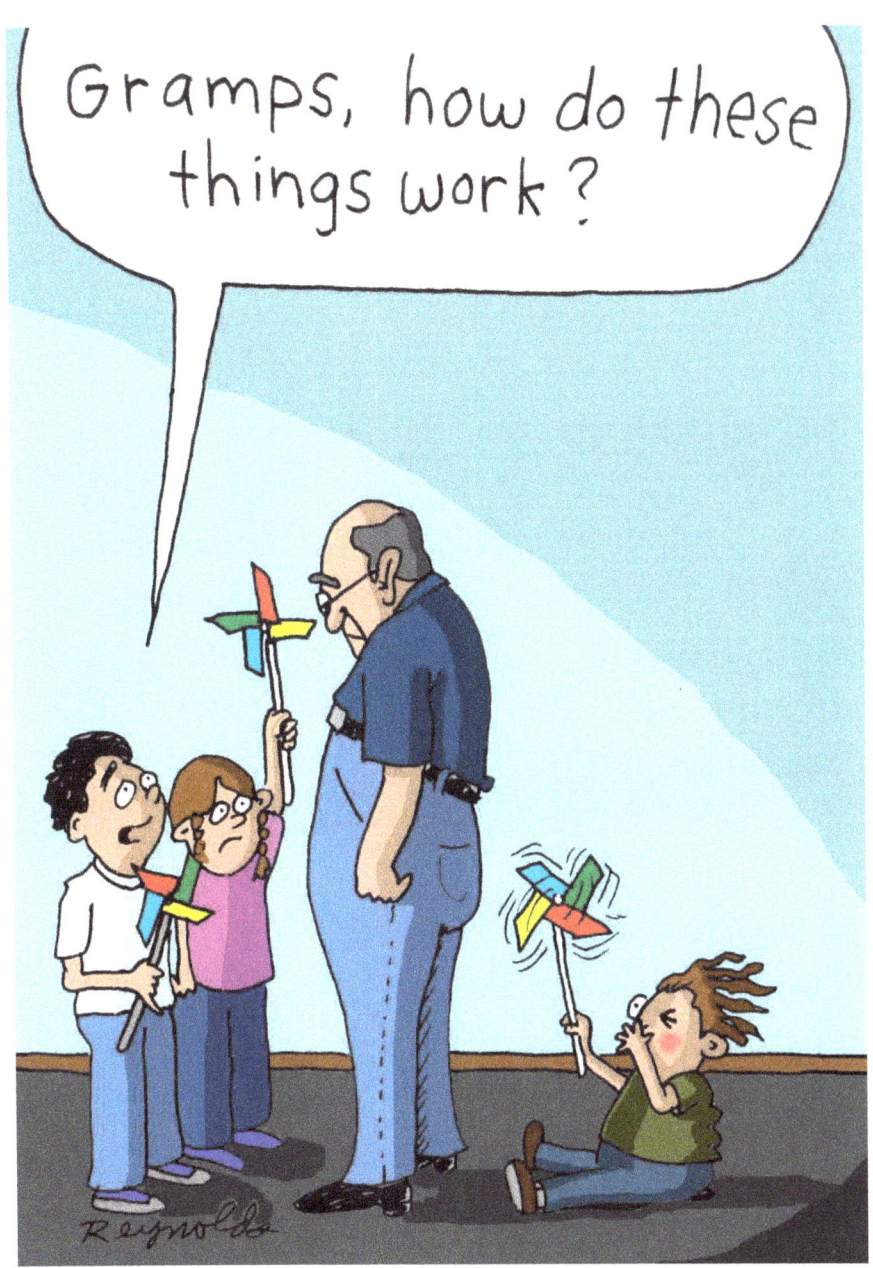

A fart travels at about ten feet per second, which works out to about seven miles per hour. It would take a fart a little more than three hours to run a standard marathon.

All the humans that have ever lived have released approximately seventeen quadrillion farts.

The Yanomami tribe who inhabit the Amazon rain forest traditionally greet one another with a loud, friendly blast of intestinal gas. The greeting has the advantage of being recognized by the hearing impaired.

A tighter anal sphincter gives rise to a louder fart. If you fart loudly you can take some pride in the fact that your anal sphincter tone is in good form.

About thirty percent of people produce flammable farts.

The Fart Side: Blowing in the Wind!

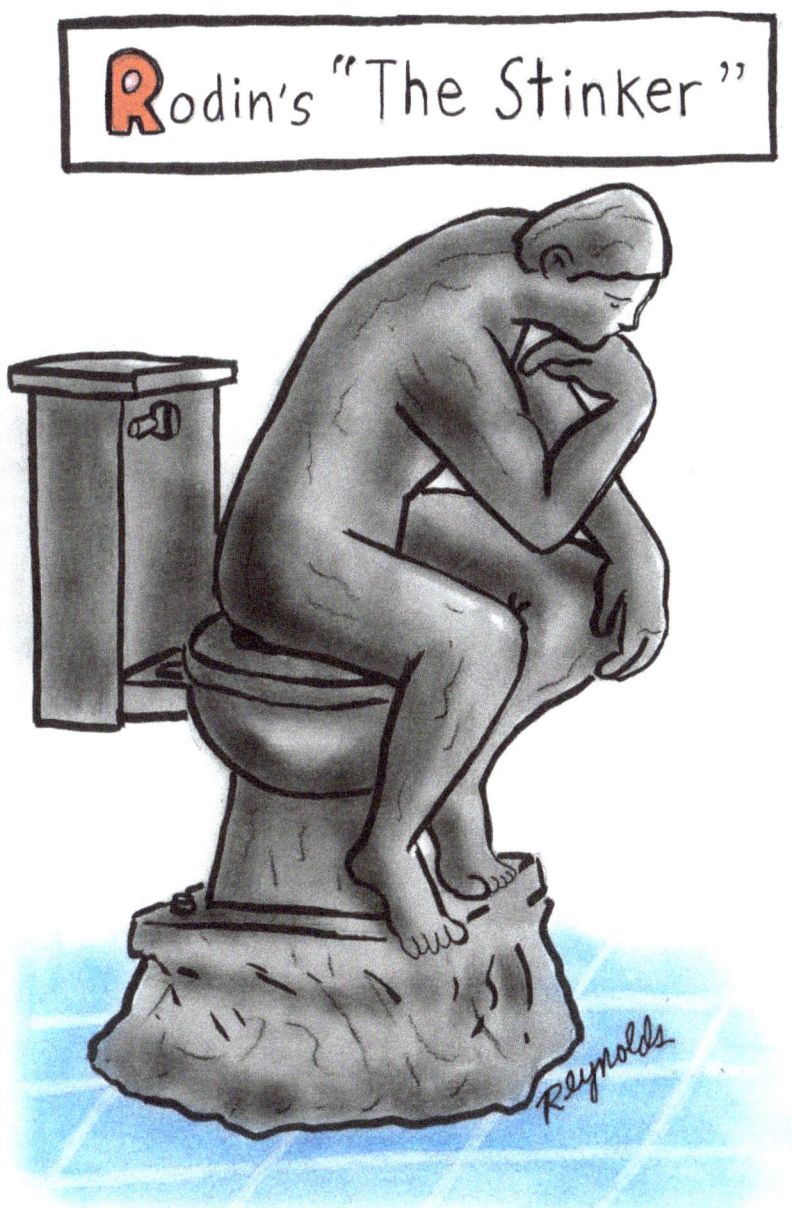

Herodotus (c.484 BCE – c425 BCE) was an ancient Greek historian, and is often referred to as the Father of History, for his classic volume *The Histories*. In the story of Apries, a fart plays a role in starting a war that killed thousands and changed the course of history.

Meals with high fat content leads to slower gut motility and transit, which allows more time for bacterial fermentation and gas production.

Hippocrates (c. 460 BCE – c. 375 BCE) was a pioneering physician who lived during Greece's Classical period, and is widely recognized as the father of modern medicine. As early as 420 B.C. Hippocrates had warned of the dangers of holding in a fart, as he wisely wrote in *Treatise on the Flatuosities*: "It is better for it to pass with noise, than to be intercepted and accumulated internally".

The Fart Side: Blowing in the Wind!

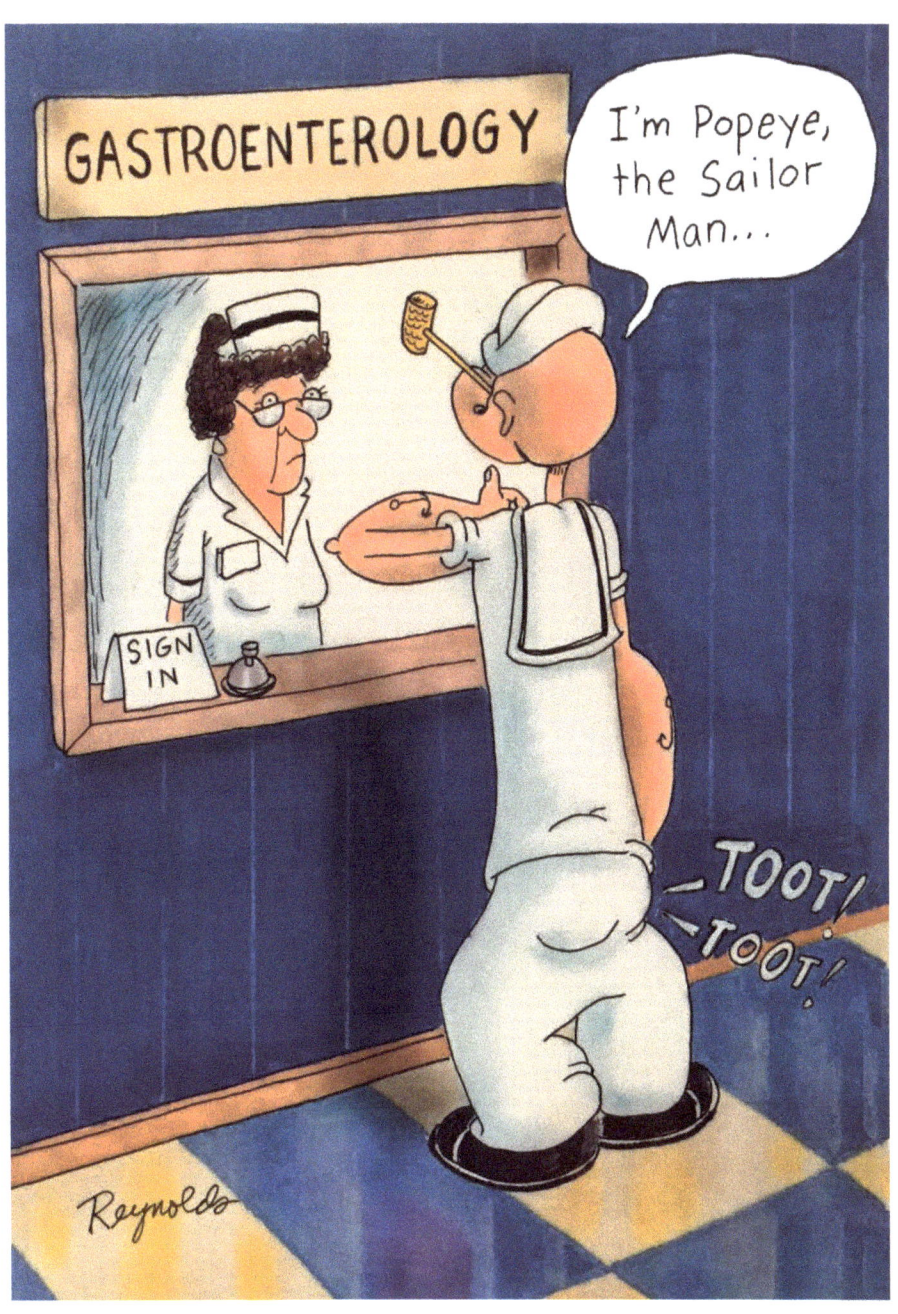

Lactose is a common additive to foods and pharmaceutical products as a filler. It may trigger symptoms in the large percentage of the human population who are lactose intolerant.

Lactose is often not clearly labeled as an ingredient in food products, and may be present as nonfat dried milk.

Hypolactasia is the formal medical term for lactose intolerance and lactase deficiency.

Every day 12 quarts (11.5 liters) of digested food, liquids and digestive juices flow through the digestive system, but only three fluid ounces (100 milliliters) are eliminated through feces.

Large quantities of carbon dioxide gas are generated when the stomach contents enter the small intestine.

The Fart Side: Blowing in the Wind!

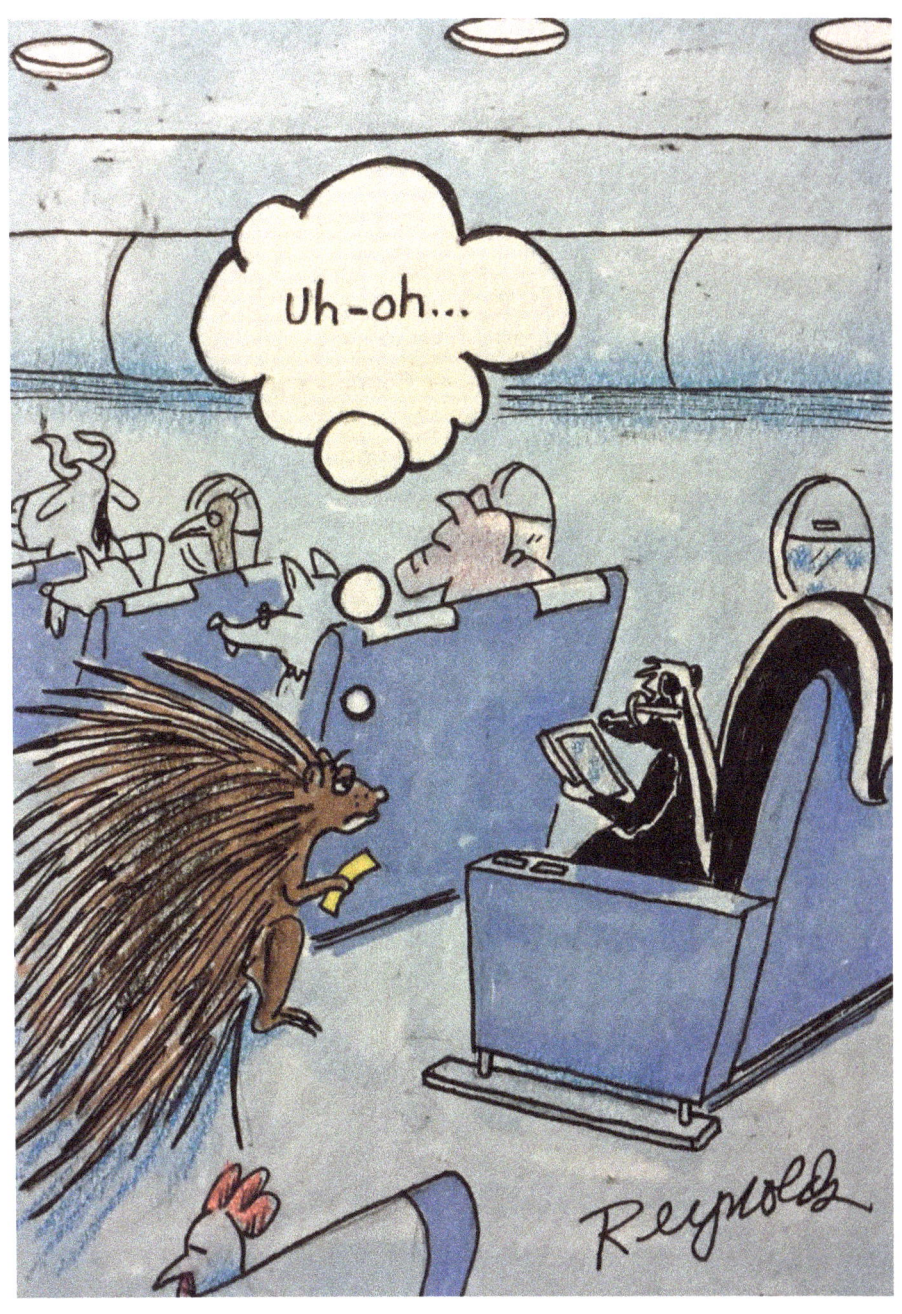

Scuba divers avoid beans and carbonated beverages before a dive because the gas bubbles in the gut can become painful on ascent.

The most common source of intestinal gas is air swallowing (aerophagia).

The average person passes more than ten farts per day.

The aroma of a fart can be an indicator of intestinal health.

Over ninety-nine percent of the gas passed in a fart is odorless.

Ice cream is often forty percent air by volume, which adds to intestinal gas.

Seventy-five percent of African-American, Jewish, Native American, and Mexican American populations are lactose intolerant.

The Fart Side: Blowing in the Wind!

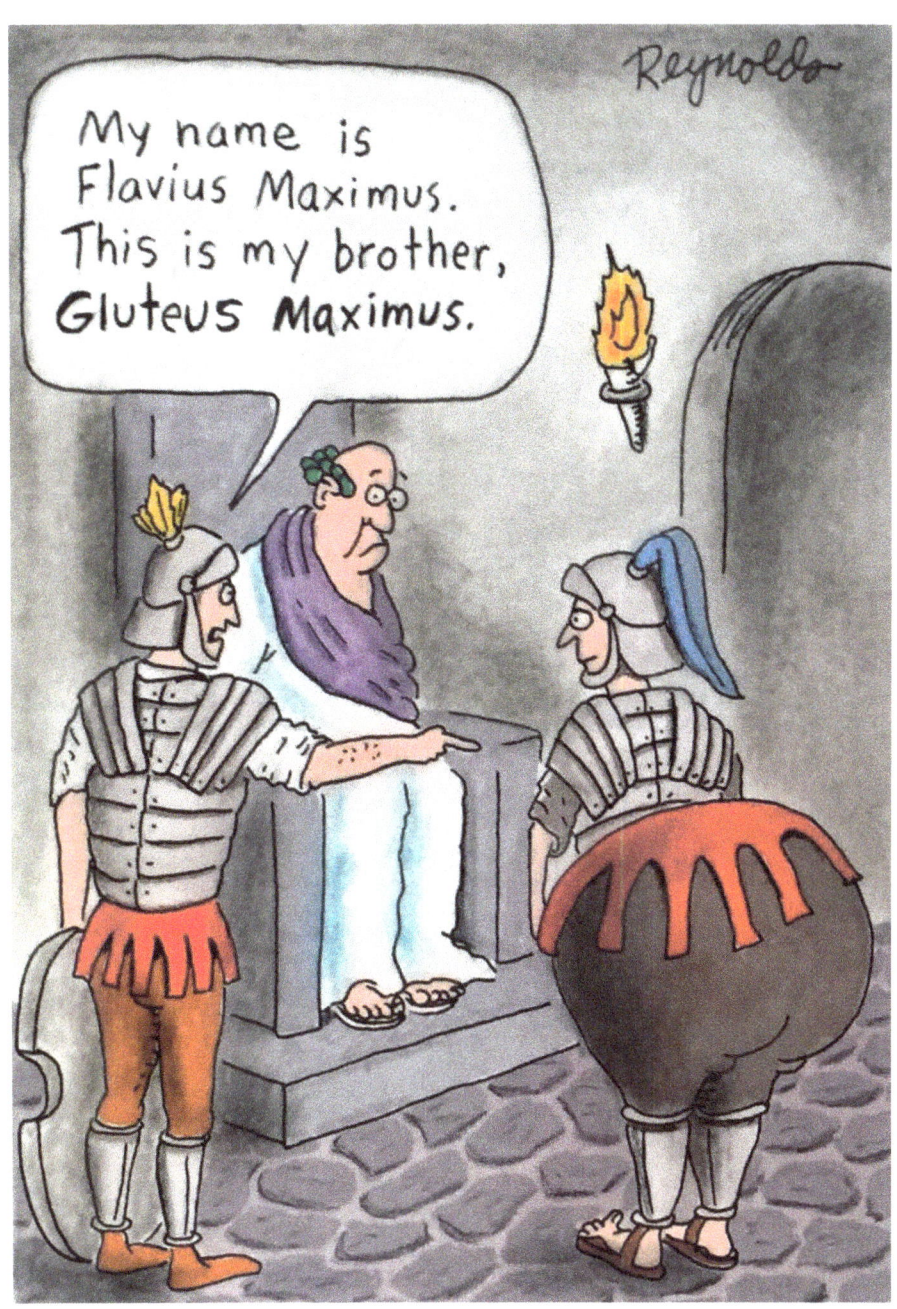

Titus Flavius Josephus (c. 37 AD – c. 100 AD) was a Roman historian during the Jewish Wars and the reign of King Herod of Judea. In *The Jewish Wars,* he describes a fart that triggered a stampede, and the deaths of twenty thousand innocent people.

Hard candy and chewing gums, which generates small volumes of saliva and frequent swallows, leads to excessive aerophagia. This air swallowing contributes to intestinal gas

Saint Jerome (c. 347 AD – 420 AD) church scholar, historian, translator, offered the following admonition: "It is good neither to eat flesh nor to drink wine – but with beans also anything that creates wind or lies heavy on the stomach should be rejected. I think that nothing so inflames the body and titillates the genitals as undigested food."

The Fart Side: Blowing in the Wind!

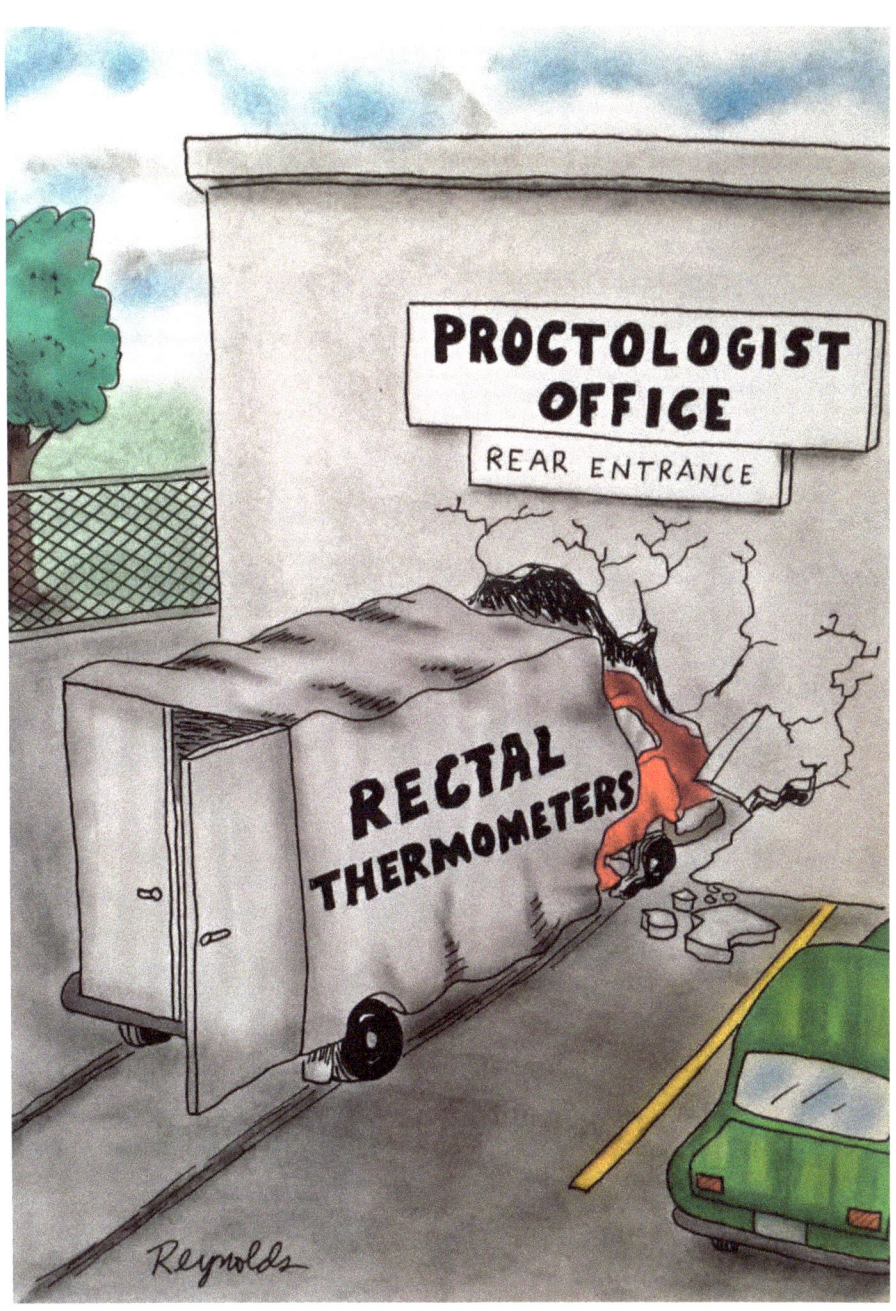

Ice cream can contribute to burping and farting, both by its air content as well as lactose intolerance.

The concept of doubling ice cream volume by mixing in air was created by Margaret Thatcher, former Prime Minister of Great Britain.

Carbonated beverages outsell dairy products by a ratio of four to one in the United States.

Carbon dioxide gas can contribute to burping and belching. It does not contribute to farting since the carbon dioxide is absorbed by the gut, enters the bloodstream, and is exhaled by the lungs.

Baby bottles are a common cause of aerophagia in infants, as they suck in and swallow air if the formula does not always cover the nipple.

The Fart Side: Blowing in the Wind!

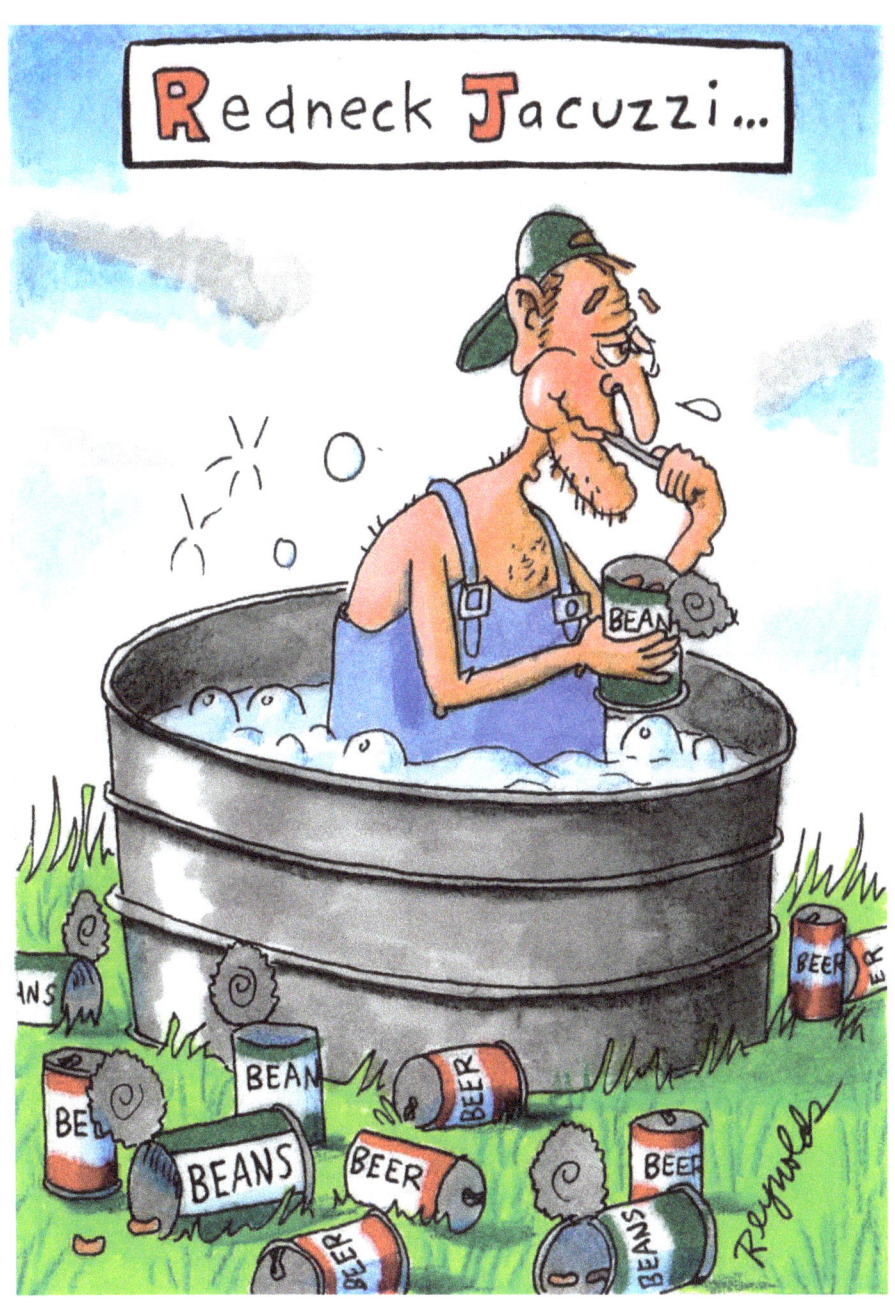

Burping the baby after a feeding is the means of allowing the swallowed air to escape, otherwise it will cause distension and discomfort.

Some bottles are designed to use an internal plastic sleeve to prevent air from reaching the nipple, when the formula is depleted the sleeve forms a vacuum so the infant is not sucking in air.

Martin Luther (1483 – 1546) was a Catholic priest and German Monk who was a major figure in the Protestant Reformation. His confrontations with the Roman Catholic Church led to his excommunication. Although a major religious figure, his published writings and letters embrace earthy bodily functions. Farting appears to be one of his favorites, and he described using his own fart production to scare off the Devil on numerous occasions.

The Fart Side: Blowing in the Wind!

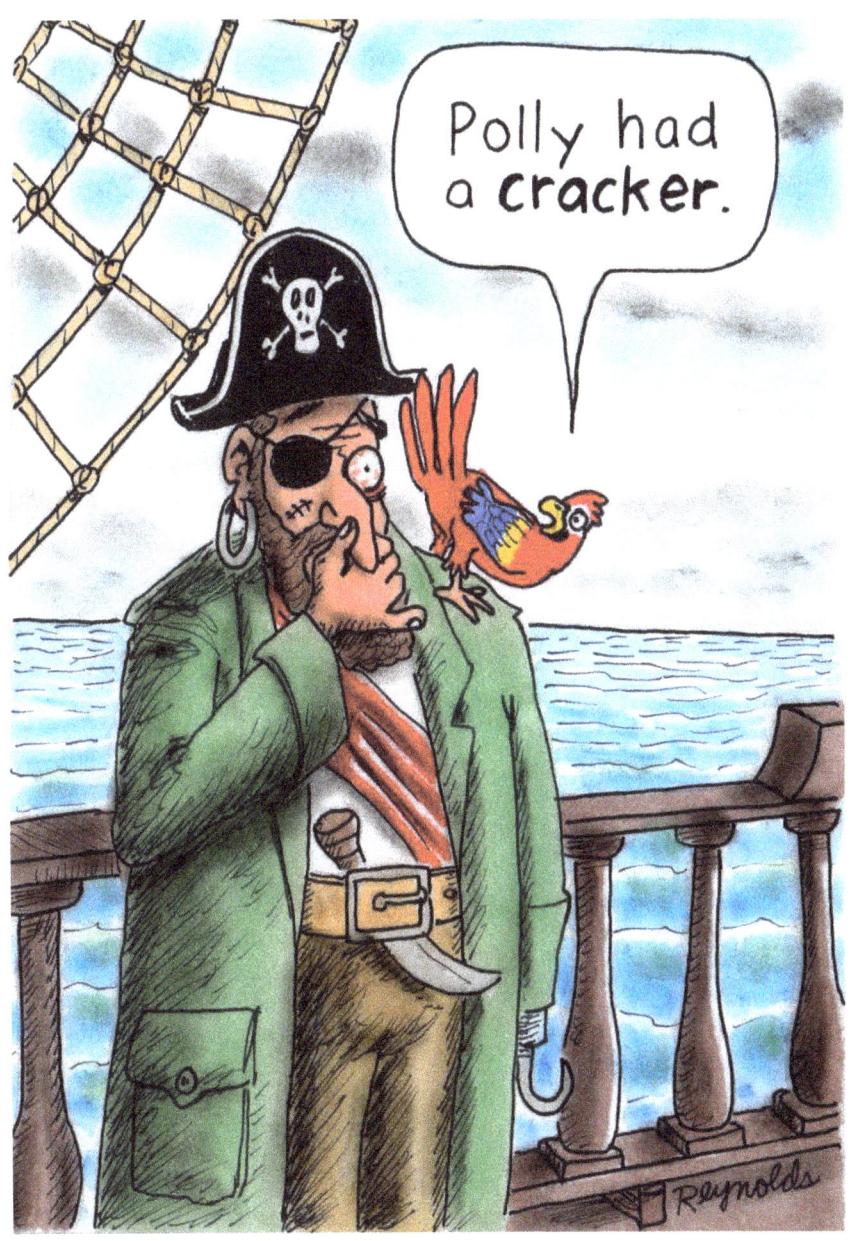

Fart travel time depends on atmospheric conditions such as wind direction, humidity, temperature, speed, the molecular weight of the fart particles including odorants and microbes, and the distance between the fart transmitter and the fart receiver.

Farts diffuse as they leave the source, and their potency diminishes with distance.

The conditions that exist for optimal fart odor concentration include when the fart is released into a small enclosed area such as an elevator, small room, car, or shower stall.

There is often a several second delay between hearing a fart and smelling it. This is due to sound traveling much more rapidly than the aroma.

The Fart Side: Blowing in the Wind!

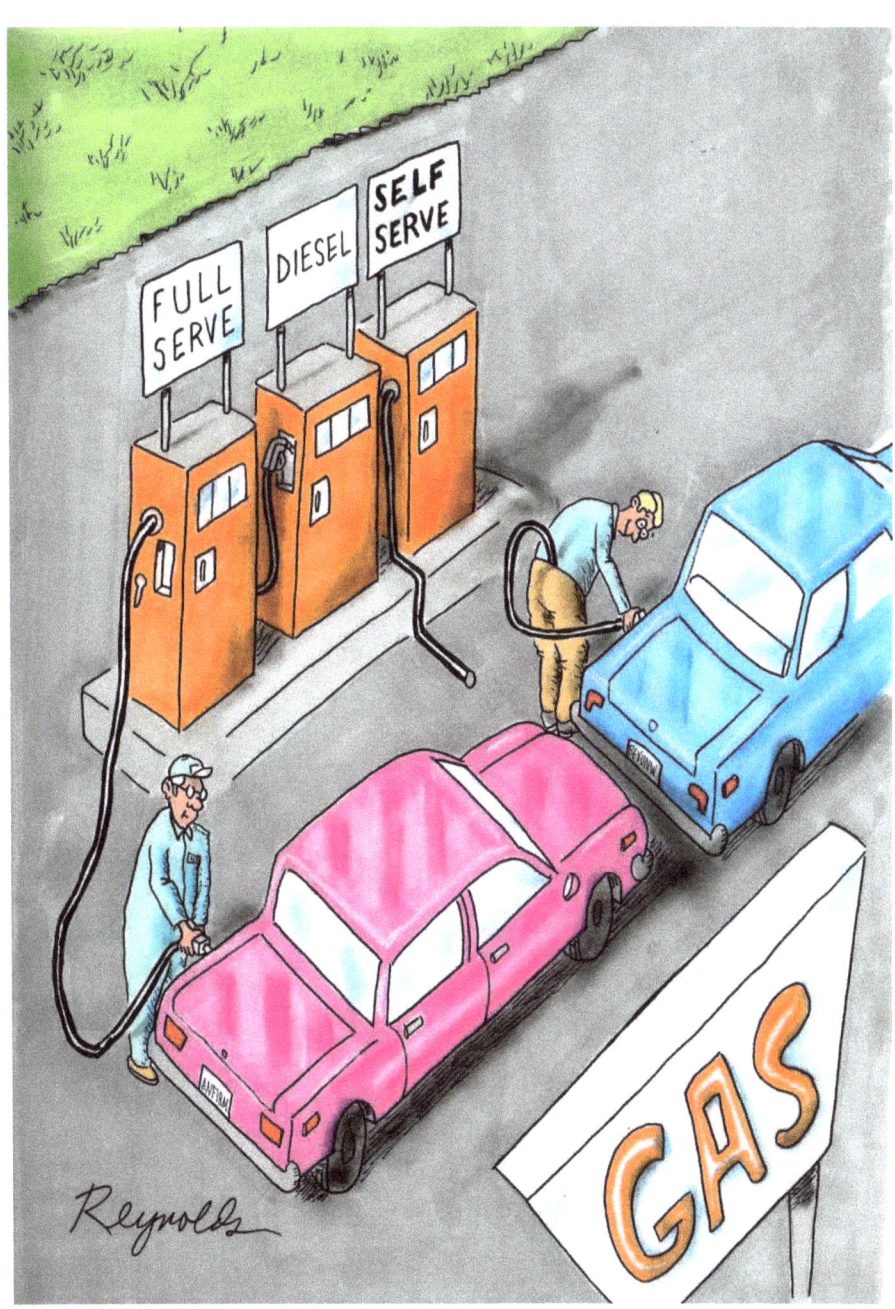

Lucius Mestrius Plutarchus (c. 46 – 120 AD) Greek historian, biographer, and essayist made the following observations about pulse and beans: "For the fruit, being new and flatulent, raises many disturbing vapors in the body."

Geoffrey Chaucer (c. 1343-1400) was a master storyteller, one of his most famous and humorous tales involving farting is that of *The Millers Wife*.

Elizabeth I (1533 – 1603) was Queen of England from 1558 until her death. The Earl of Oxford, was required to curtsy before Her Majesty the Queen, as per court protocol. As the portly Earl curtsied, he accidently released a loud fart. He was so embarrassed that he went into exile from the royal court for ten years. When he returned Queen Elizabeth offered a sly pardon and said, 'My Lord, I hath forgot the fart".

The Fart Side: Blowing in the Wind!

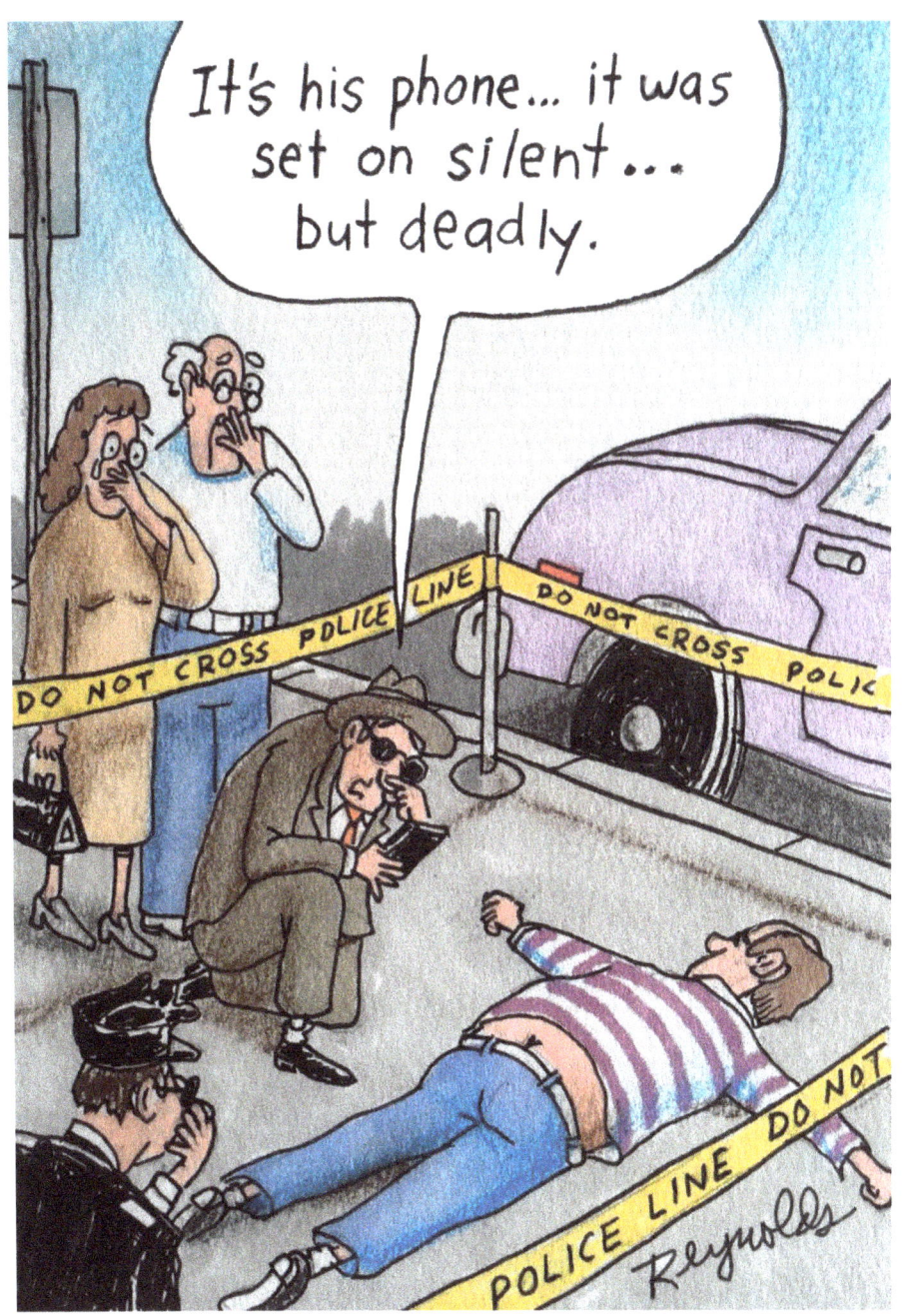

It is possible to capture a fart in a sealed container. To capture a fart bubble underwater, release it into a water filled jar held upside down. To properly preserve the fart, avoid any reaction of sulfur based gasses with glass, plastic, or rubber. The container should be made of pure polypropylene.

The female southern pine beetle releases a pheromone, a hormone that serves as an olfactory sexual attractant, called frontalin in her flatus. It serves to attract males, but also attracts other females to engage with the males who respond. Predators are also attracted by the pheromone, recognizing that it will lead to more prey.

Seventy-eight percent of air is nitrogen. The gastrointestinal tract poorly absorbs this gas compared to oxygen, hydrogen, and carbon dioxide.

The Fart Side: Blowing in the Wind!

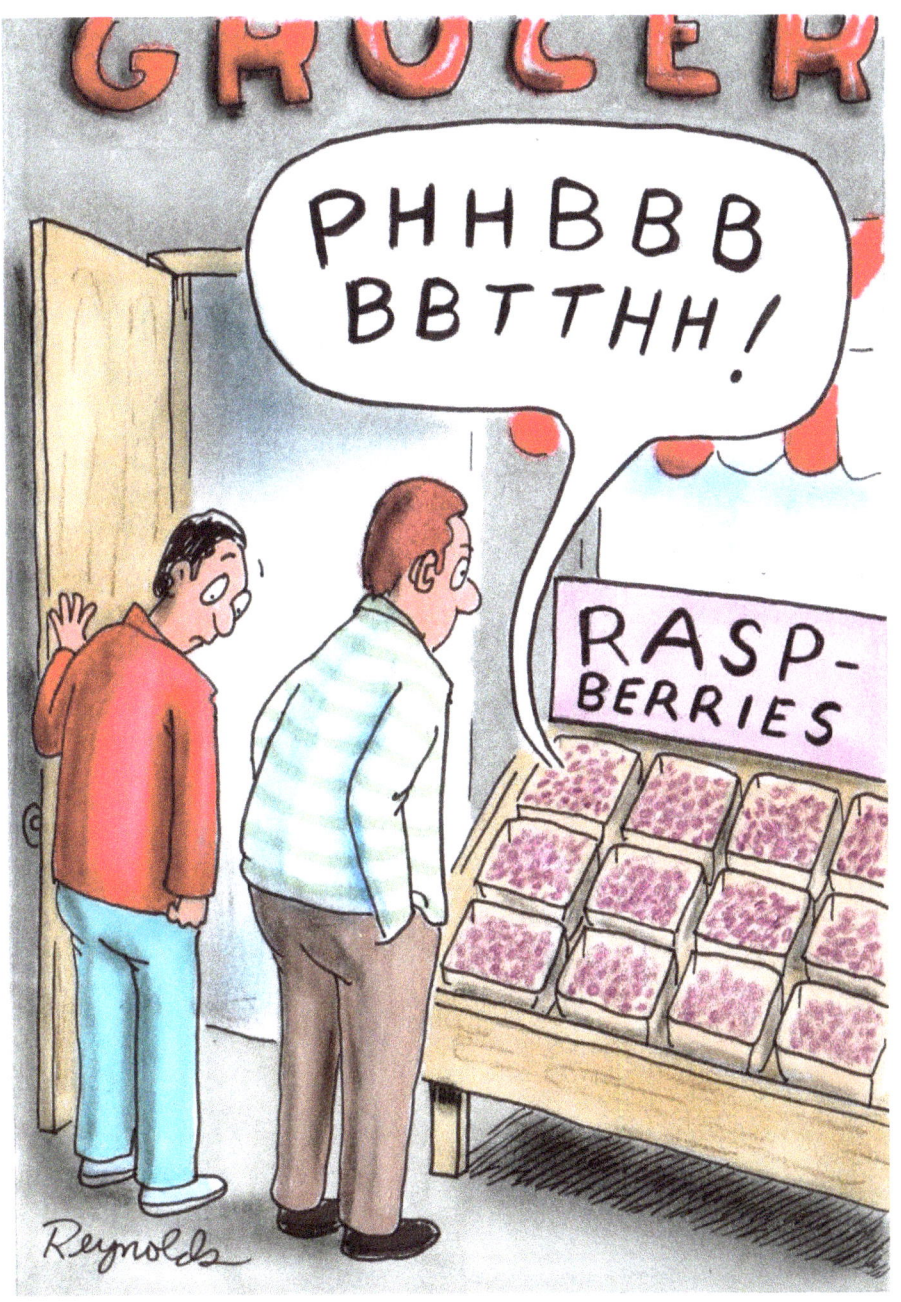

The surface area of the human digestive tract exceeds that of a championship tennis court.

Henry Ludlow (1577–1639), a Member of Parliament in England was participating in a vigorous debate. When the roll call for votes took place, it was his turn to respond and everyone expected him to offer a resounding NAY! Which he did in the form of a loud fart.

Oliver Cromwell (1599-1658) was a controversial English leader who has been variously labeled as a regicide, dictator, and hero of liberty. Cromwell's derogatory response to a critic quoting the Magna Carta was "I care not for the Magna Farta".

Farts are ubiquitous, all living creatures generate gas from cellular metabolism and respiration.

The Fart Side: Blowing in the Wind!

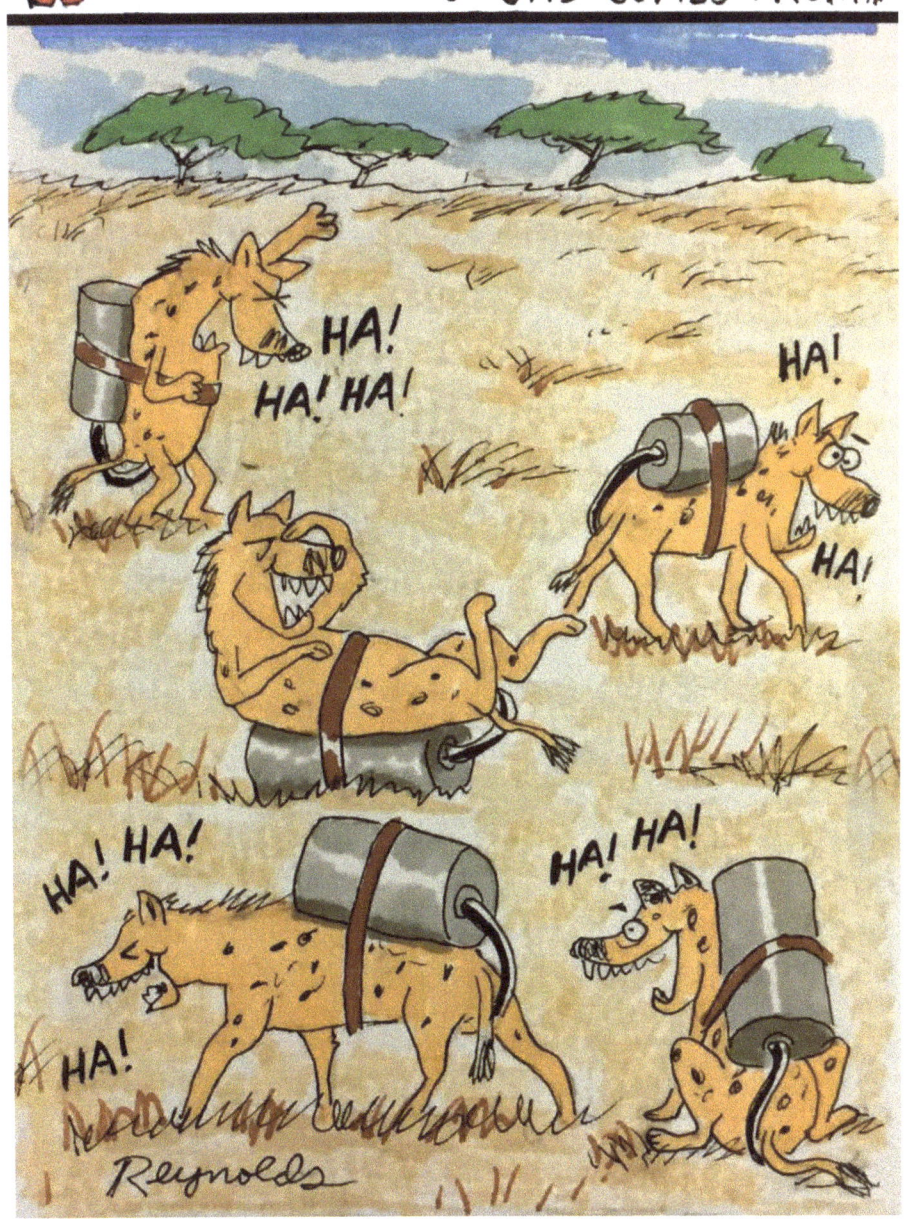

Termites are a major contributor to greenhouse gasses and global warming. They comprise a large portion of the world's biomass, and the microbes in their intestinal tract metabolize the cellulose in the wood they eat, releasing large quantities of methane.

Depending on herd and population size cows, pigs, sheep, horses, dogs, cats, kangaroos, camels, zebras, elephants, and other animals are also major contributors to global warming by farting and belching methane.

If you fart consistently for six years and nine months, enough gas is produced to create the energy of a small atomic bomb.

Digestive enzymes are secreted in the saliva, mouth, stomach, pancreas, small intestine, and gut microbiome.

The Fart Side: Blowing in the Wind!

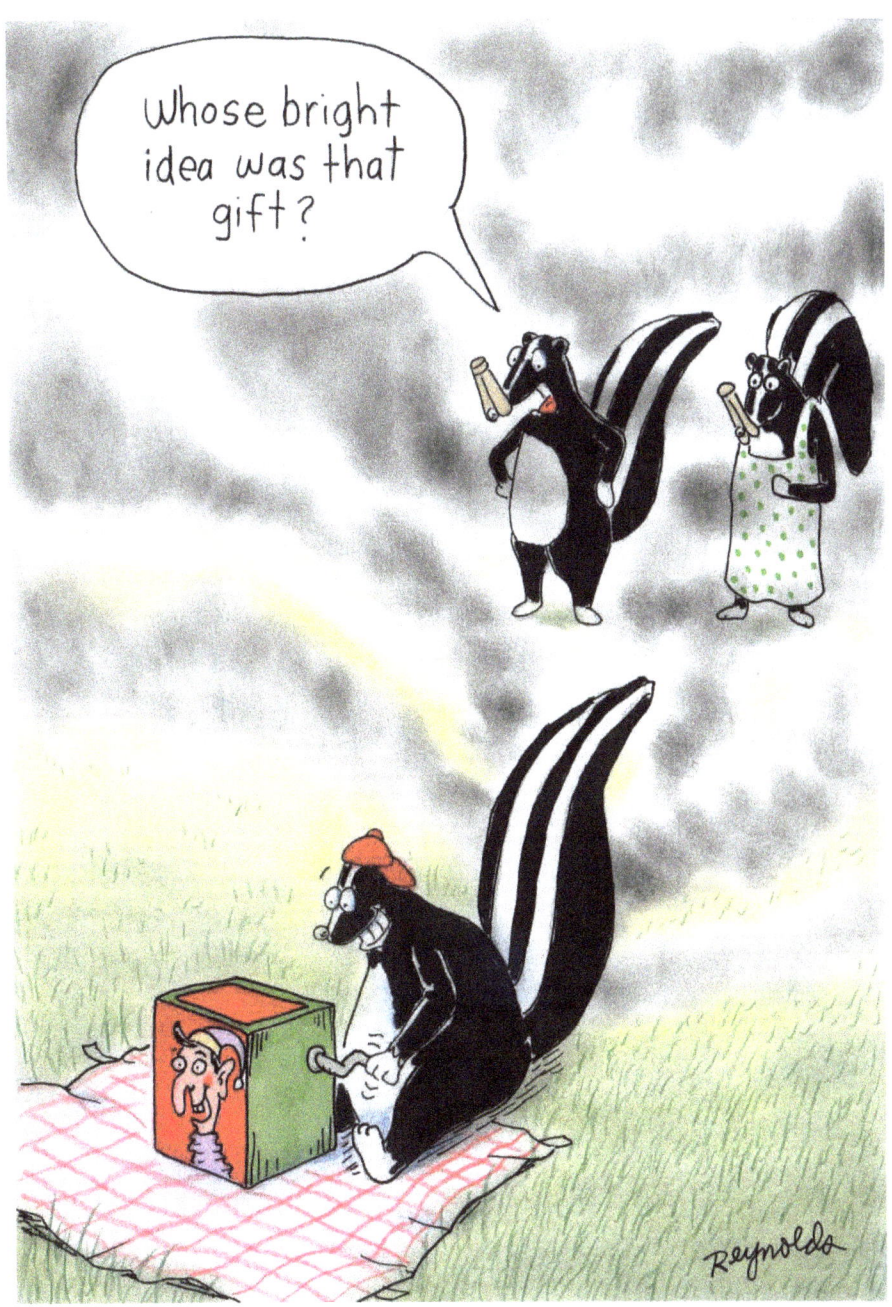

Adolf Hitler (1889 – 1945) was the Austrian born Chancellor of Germany, and dictator (Führer) of Nazi Germany during WWII. According to Pulitzer Prize winning historian and biographer John Toland, Hitler "suffered from meteorism, uncontrollable farting".

About thirty percent of people enjoy the aroma of their farts.

The liver is the only organ in the human body that can regenerate itself completely.

Josef Stalin (1878-1953) ruled the Soviet Union with an iron fist from the mid-1920s until his death in 1953. Stalin had a profound phobia of farting in public. When attending meetings, he would have two water glasses that he would clink together repeatedly, to mask the sound of his farts.

The Fart Side: Blowing in the Wind!

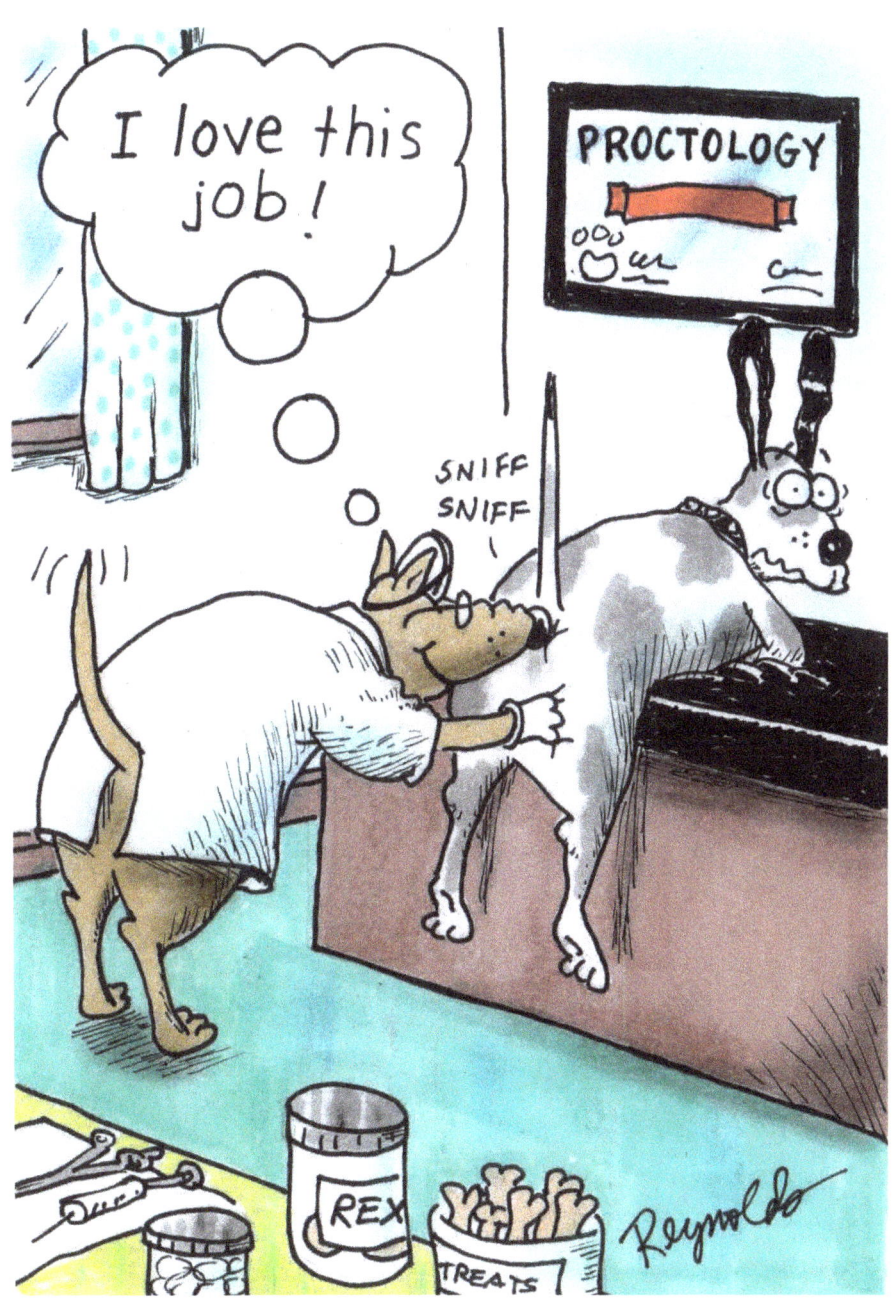

Enzyme supplements to reduce gas from beans and legumes can be very effective.

Air is seventy-eight percent nitrogen, which is poorly absorbed by the gut, and contributes to burping and farts.

Sipping smaller volumes increases the amount of air swallowed (aerophagia), and contributes to burping and farts.

The average person swallows two thousand times per day, and each swallow includes five milliliters (one teaspoon) of air.

The average person swallows every thirty seconds while awake, and every five minutes while asleep.

The calories you burn simply digesting food account for up to fifteen percent of your energy expenditure.

The Fart Side: Blowing in the Wind!

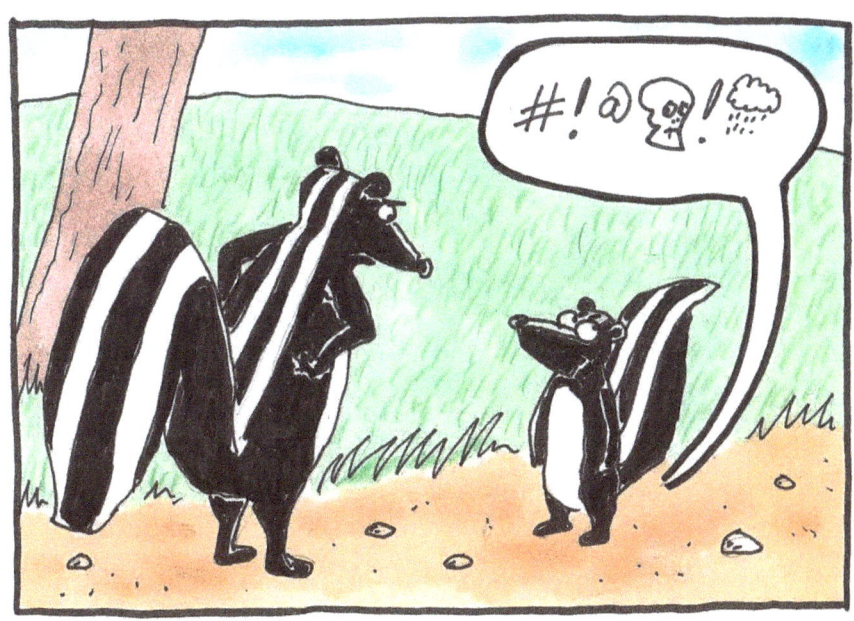

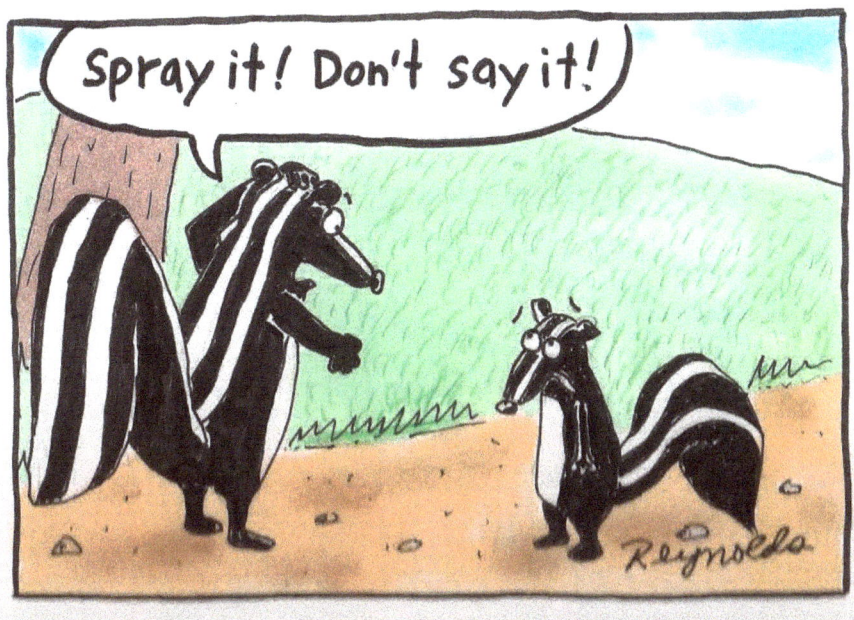

The Great Chicago Fire which destroyed the city in 1871 has traditionally been blamed on Mrs. O'Leary's cow kicking over a kerosene lamp. With the large volume of methane produced by the average cow, it is just as likely to have been caused by her cow farting and belching.

It takes around six hours for the average human to digest a meal that is high in fat content. A meal rich in carbohydrates, on the other hand, takes around two hours to digest.

Gaius Petronius Arbiter (c. 27 – 66 AD) was a Roman courtier during the reign of Nero. He is the author of *Satyricon*, a satirical novel. "Take my word for it, friends, the vapors go straight to your brain. Poison your whole system. I know some who have died from being too polite and holding it in", referring to unreleased farts.

The Fart Side: Blowing in the Wind!

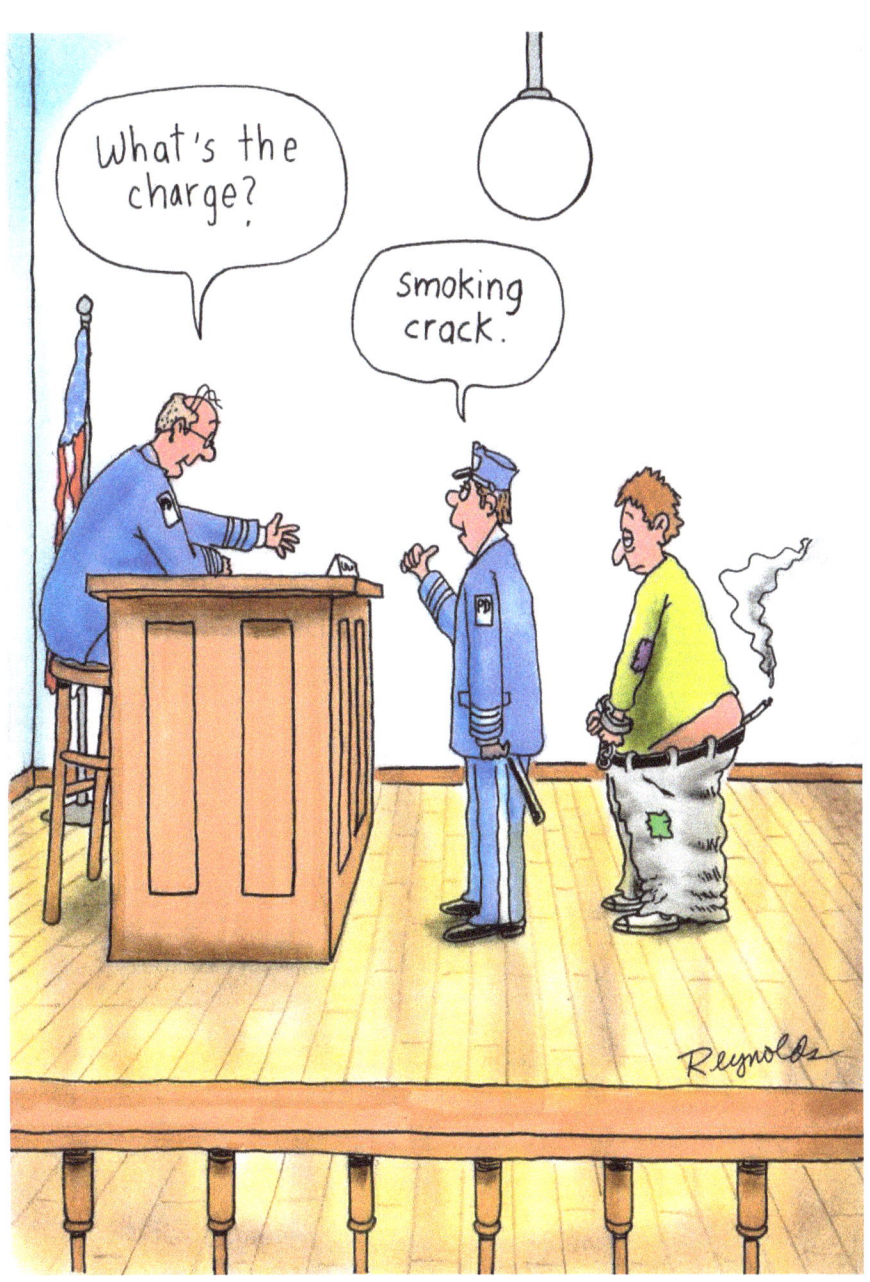

SCUBA divers cannot fart at depths of thirty-three feet or below. This is because the high atmospheric pressure exceeds the pressure needed to expel the gas.

Jonathan Swift (1667 – 1745) was an Anglo-Irish author, essayist, satirist, and cleric. The pamphlet *The Benefit of Farting Explained* was published under his puffed-up pseudonym of Don Fartinando Puff-Indorst, Professor of Bumbast at the University of Crackow.

Samuel Langhorne Clemens (1835 - 1910), under the pen name Mark Twain, was one of America's most famous authors and humorists. His short story *1601* is a ribald work about farting at the Royal Court of Queen Elizabeth I of Great Britain.

The stomach produces hydrochloric acid, which kills many microbes.

The Fart Side: Blowing in the Wind!

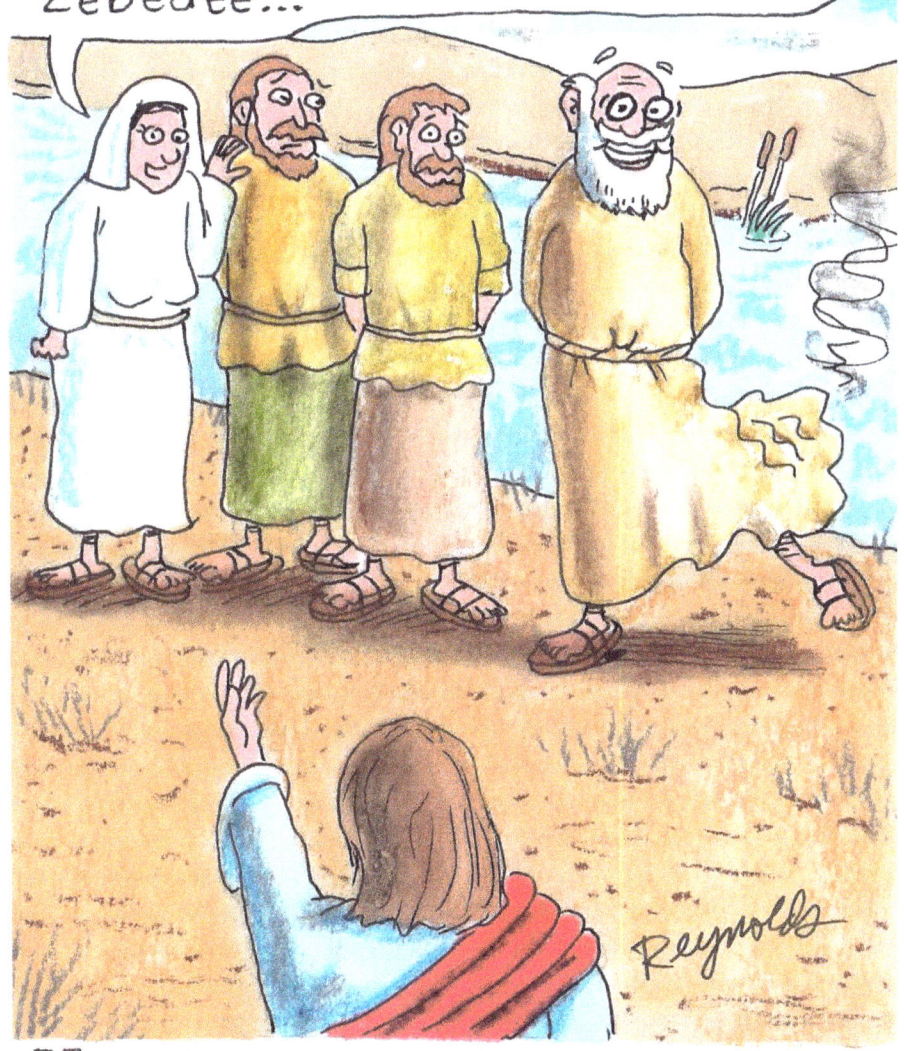

Roald Dahl (1916-1990) was an English novelist, poet, and fighter pilot who became one of the 20th century's favorite authors of children's books. In *The BFG* the character The Big Friendly Giant engages in an activity described as whizzpopping, the passing of intestinal gas, at formal events. The giants believe burps are disgusting, but farts are entertaining and they love farting.

The Russian words for fart include *perdyozh* (first act of breaking wind), *perdun* (perpetrator and outcome), *perdil'nik* (place from where it comes), *Perun* (ancient God of wind), *bzdun* (silent fart), and bzdyukha (silent fart, as well as a stupid jerk).

The hydrochloric acid in the stomach provides an optimum pH for the activation and reaction of enzymes.

The Fart Side: Blowing in the Wind!

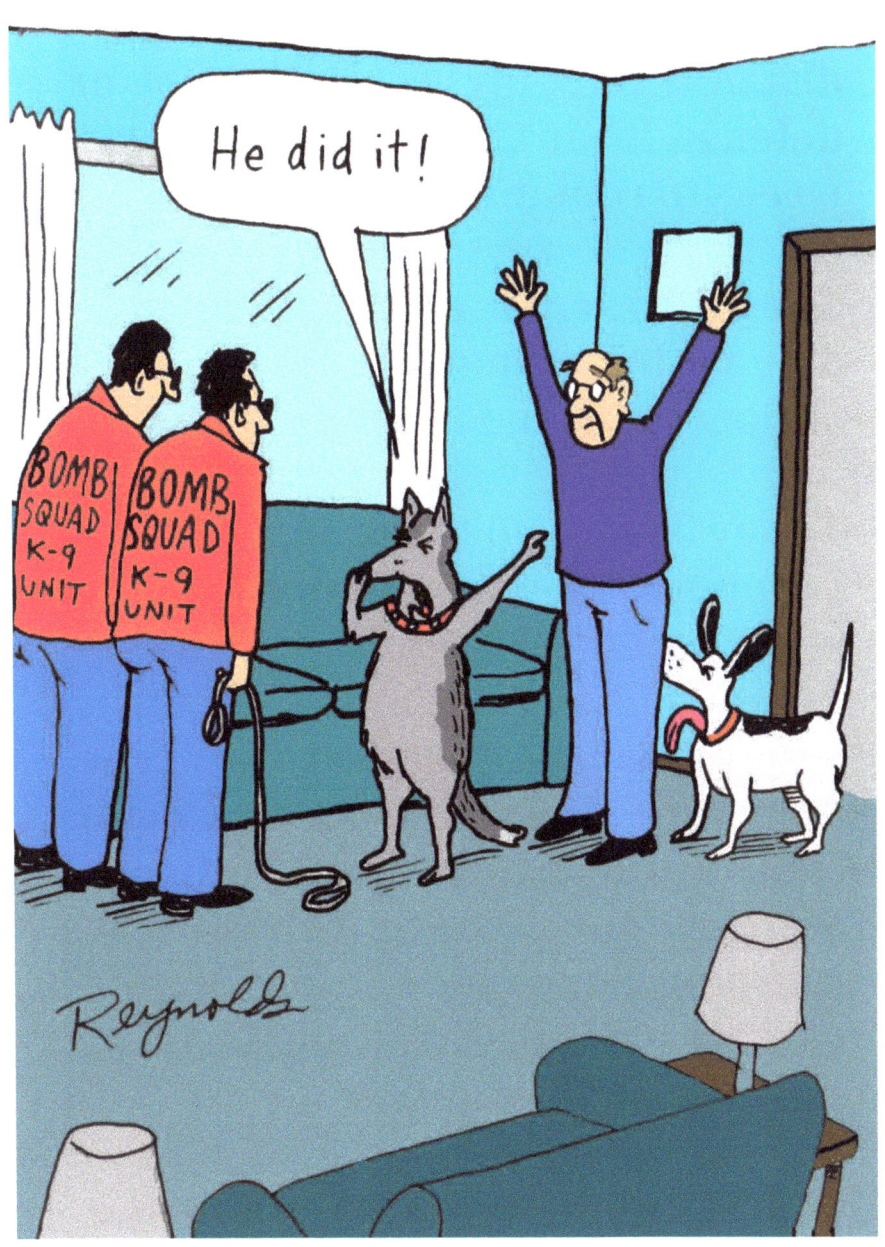

Skunks release the contents of their anal glands over a ten-foot spray distance, but only as a last resort for defense. It can take them up to two weeks to replenish their supply.

The saliva serves as a first line of defense in our immune system. It has antibacterial and immune properties.

To say fart in *American Sign Language:* The non-dominant hand is an "A" or an "S" handshape. The dominant hand is a bent hand and is held so that the fingers are underneath the pinkie side of the non-dominant "fist." The dominant hand "unbends" and bends one time as if showing gas escaping. For comic effect or emphasis, you can puff one cheek and force a bit of air through your lips.

Over four billion people around the world never use toilet paper.

The Fart Side: Blowing in the Wind!

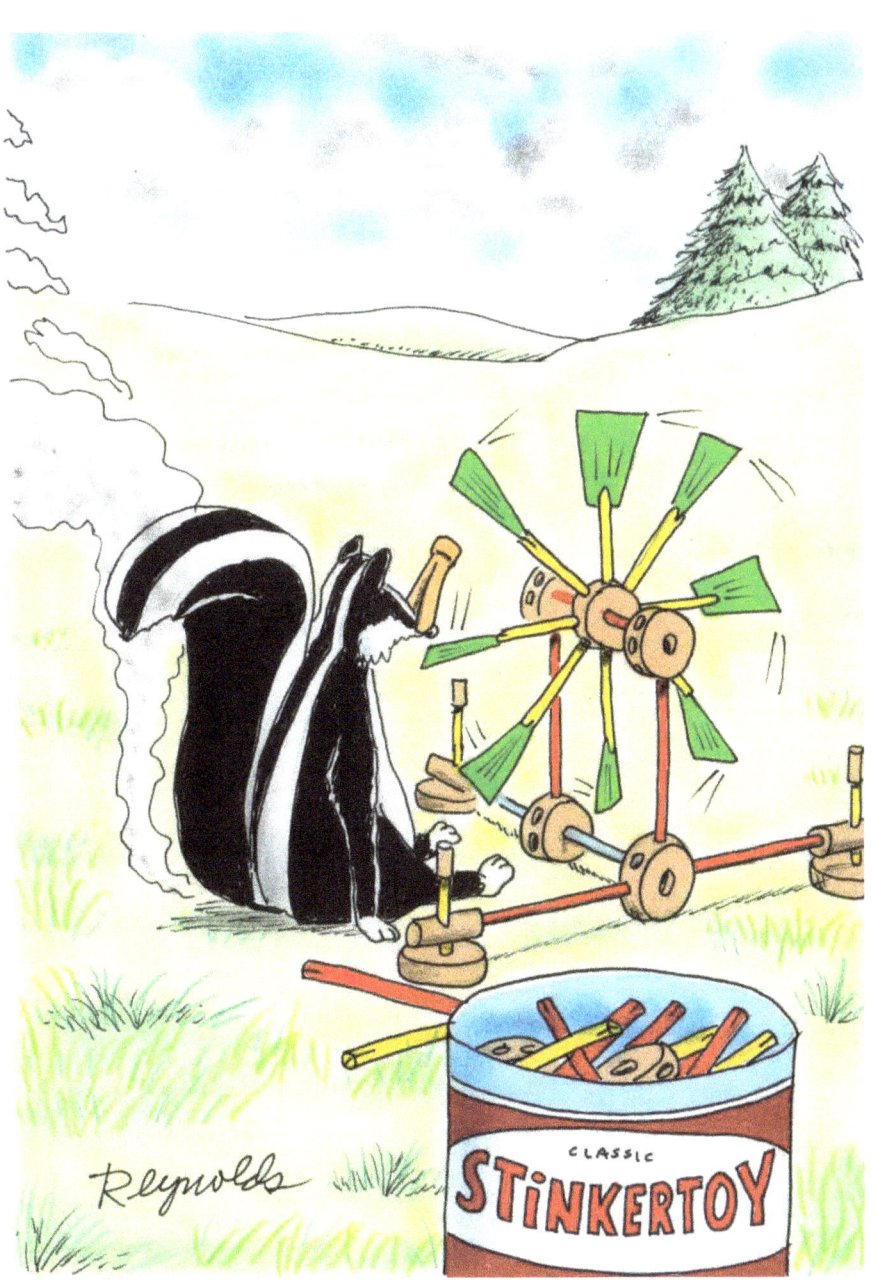

Nearly thirty thousand trees a day are harvested and converted into toilet paper.

The diversity of the English vocabulary is due to its history of occupation by foreigners, especially during the days of the Roman Empire. The Romans did not impose their own language, in this case Latin, on the inhabitants of the British Isles. The population adapted their native tongue to include words borrowed from the occupiers and foreign influences. This led to the rapid expansion of the English vocabulary, including many different words that are synonyms.

In ancient Japan, public contests were held to see who could fart the loudest and longest.

Twenty million Americans suffer from chronic digestive diseases.

The Fart Side: Blowing in the Wind!

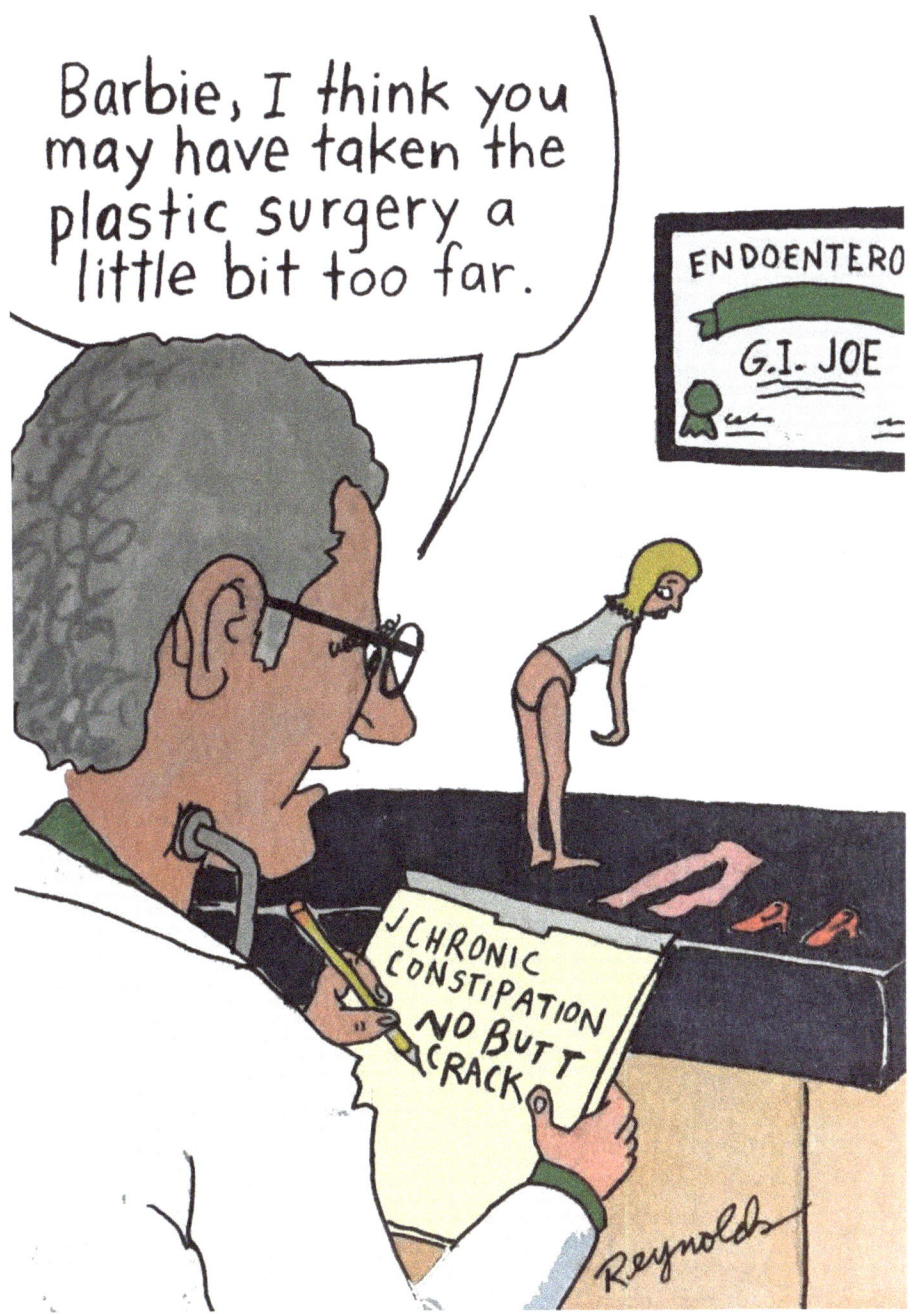

Farts are ubiquitous, as all living creatures generate gas from cellular metabolism and respiration. Humans are no exception, and can even fart for a period after death.

The natural gas methane is odorless.

As the gut microbiome metabolizes fiber and prebiotics it generates vast quantities of gases. Among these gaseous products are odiferous hydrogen sulfide, which has a foul smell like a rotten egg.

Other gases that contribute to the characteristic fecal odor include indole, skatole, ammonia, and mercaptans. They commonly arise with the digestion of tryptophan, animal proteins, and fats.

In low concentration indole has a flowery perfume smell.

The Fart Side: Blowing in the Wind!

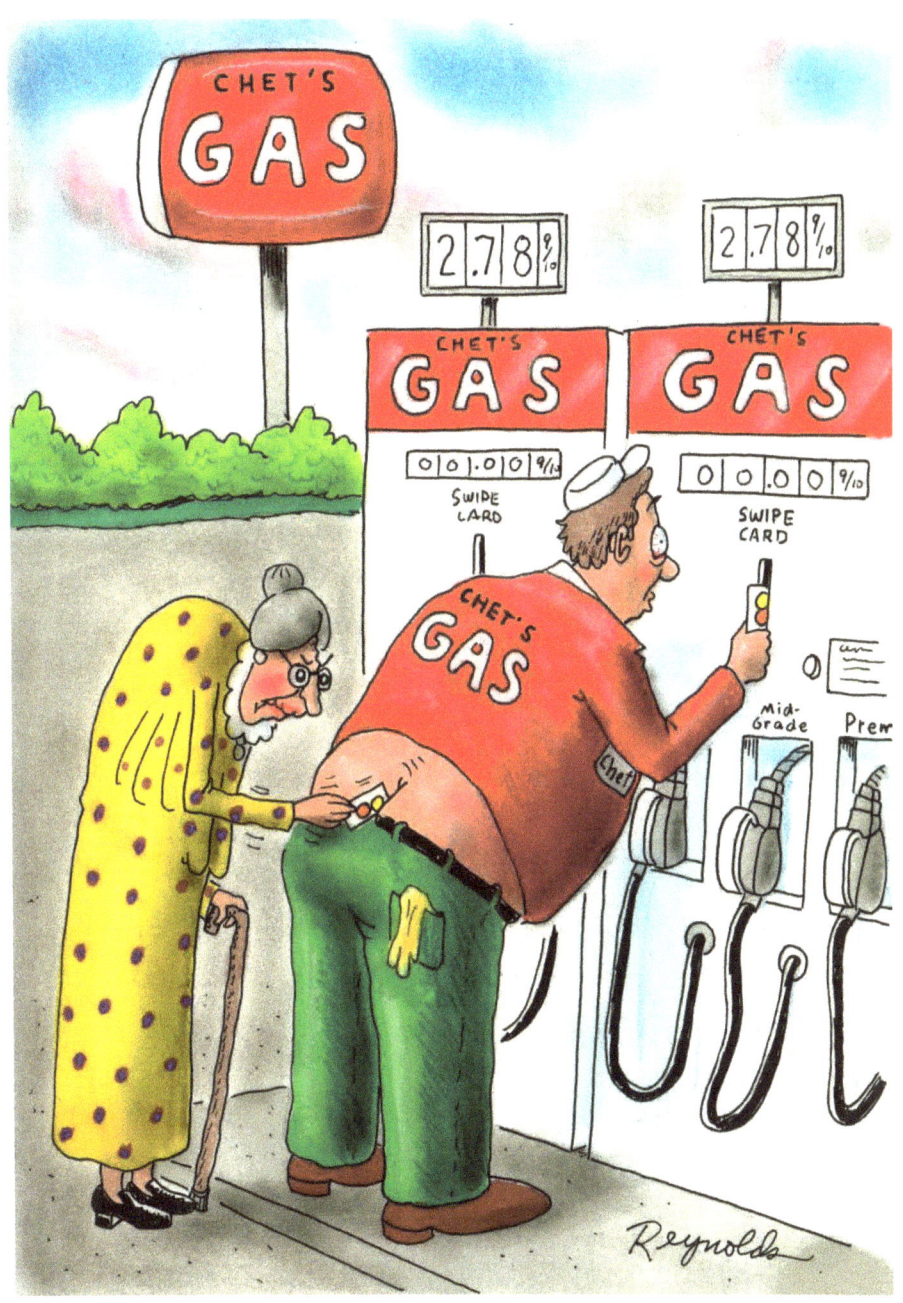

It took extensive scientific study to collect the intestinal gasses of herds of cattle before a startling discovery was made. Scientists were surprised that the clear majority of the methane production was coming from the stomach end of the cows and other ruminants, not their rear ends. It is the burps and belches arising from the multi-compartment ruminant stomach, where microbial fermentation takes place, that is the primary source of methane.

Termites, which have over two thousand species, produce twenty-five percent of the methane contributing to global warming. Technically, it is the microbes in their guts that produces the methane.

More Americans are hospitalized with digestive diseases than any other type of disorder.

The Fart Side: Blowing in the Wind!

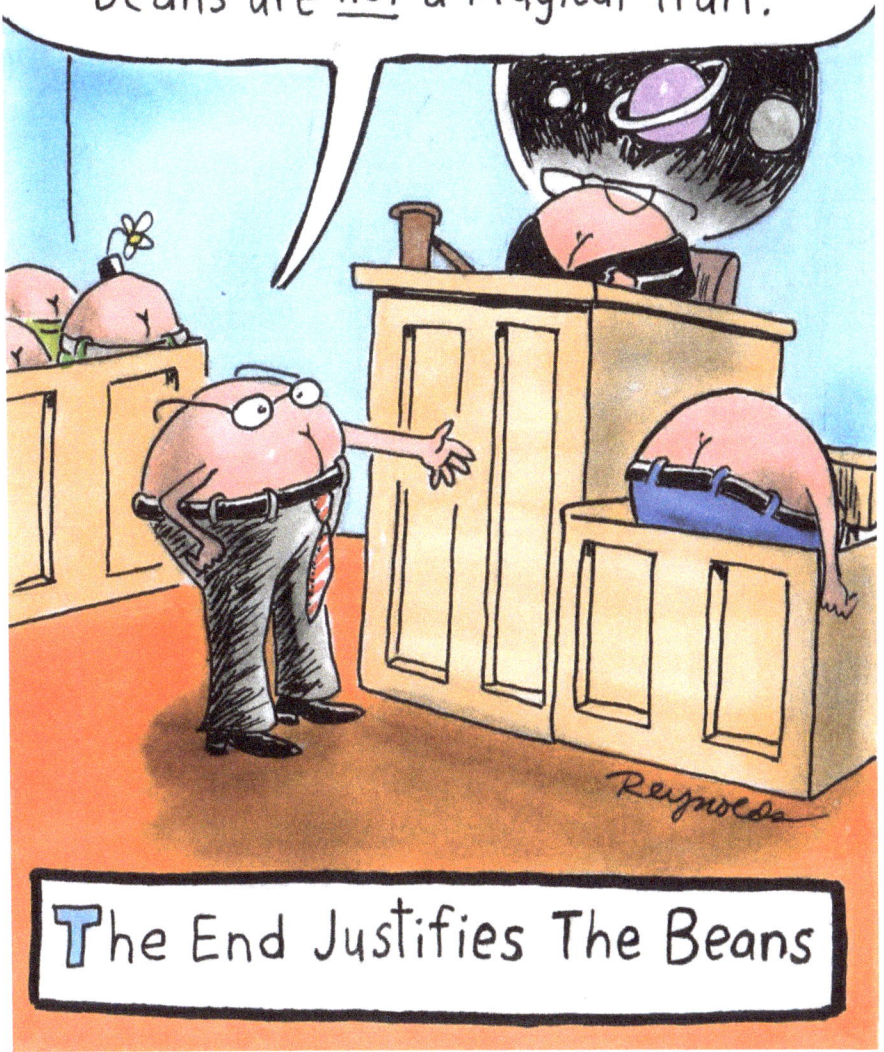

Ruminant bacterial fermentation is a significant contributor to global methane production.

Methane is over twenty times as potent as carbon dioxide as a greenhouse gas.

To reduce livestock methane production, several countries have proposed taxes on the herds responsible for the release of the gas.

Atlantic herring fish communicate distress signals to the rest of the school of fish by farting.

Skatole, which has the characteristic odor of feces, is attractive to males of various species of bees and mosquitos.

The parietal cells of the stomach secrete a glycoprotein called intrinsic factor which enables the absorption of vitamin B-12.

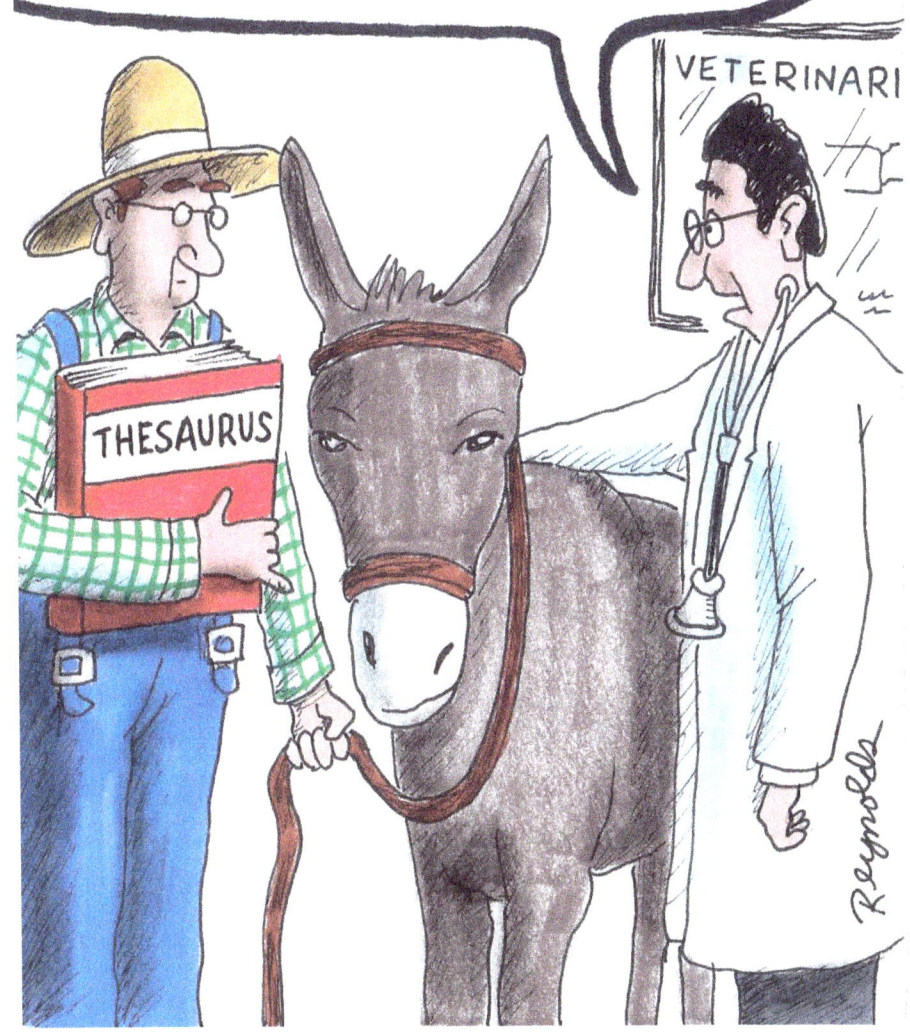

Dinosaurs have been accused of contributing to global warming. It is not known if they were ruminants, but there is no doubt that they were major farters. Their nickname "thunder lizards" may have more to do with their farts, than their footsteps.

Some dog breeds fart more than others, especially the short snouted English bulldog, and similar breeds that are regular air swallowers. Lap dogs were specifically bred to be small enough for a lady to always keep with her, and if intestinal gas ruffled her undergarments, she would simply blame her readily available dog for the emission.

Digestive diseases represent one of the US most serious health problems in terms of discomfort and pain, personal expenditures for treatment, working hours lost, and mortality.

The Fart Side: Blowing in the Wind!

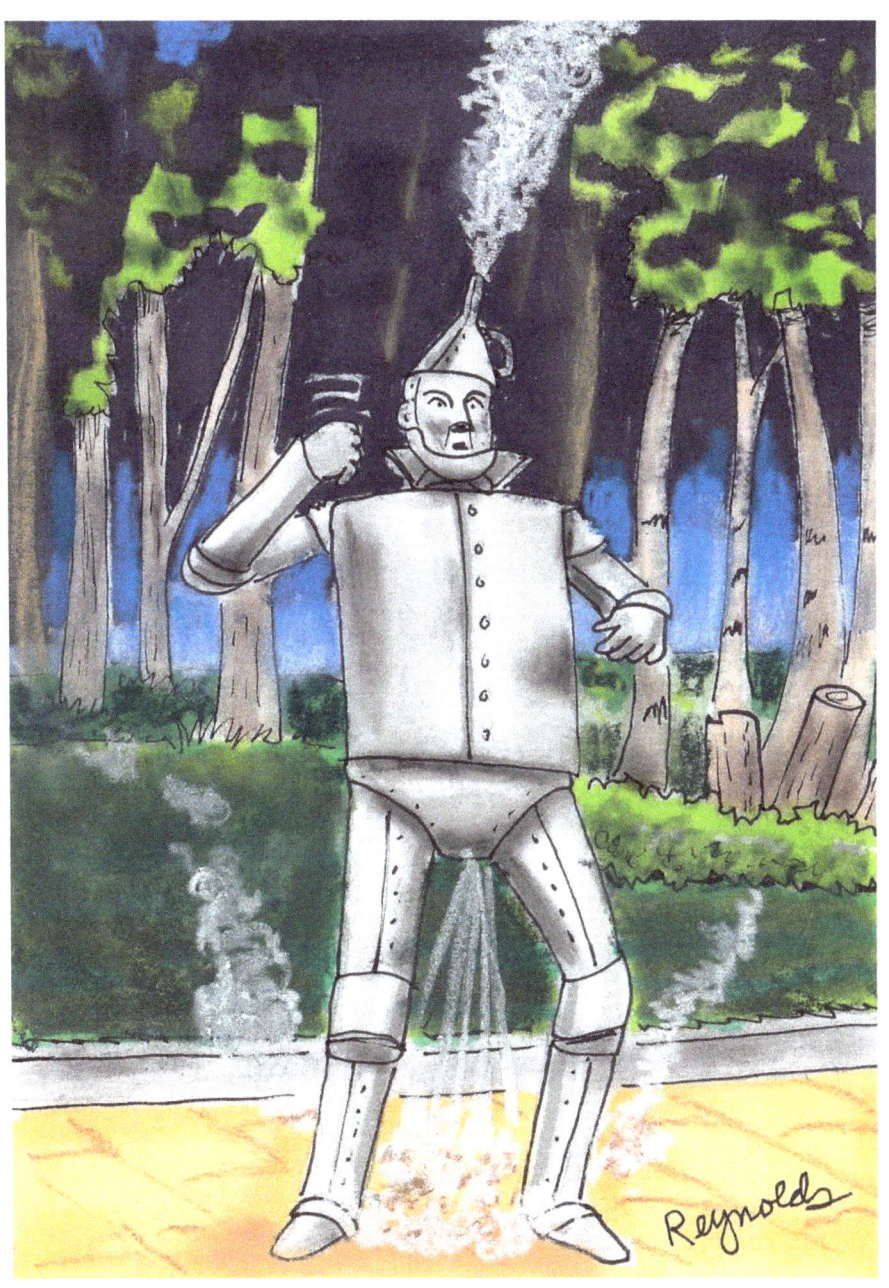

One third of Americans flush while still sitting on the toilet. This is very dangerous on aircraft and cruise ships where a powerful vacuum flush can lead to severe internal injuries if a tight seal occurs with sitting.

There are forty thousand injuries a year while sitting on the toilet seat.

Termites trapped in amber, the petrified sap of trees, have preserved pockets of gas that still contain the methane that the termites passed hundreds to thousands of years ago.

An average cow is thought to release about six hundred liters (one hundred and sixty gallons) of methane per day through burping.

Fourteen million cases of acute digestive diseases are treated in the United States each year.

The Fart Side: Blowing in the Wind!

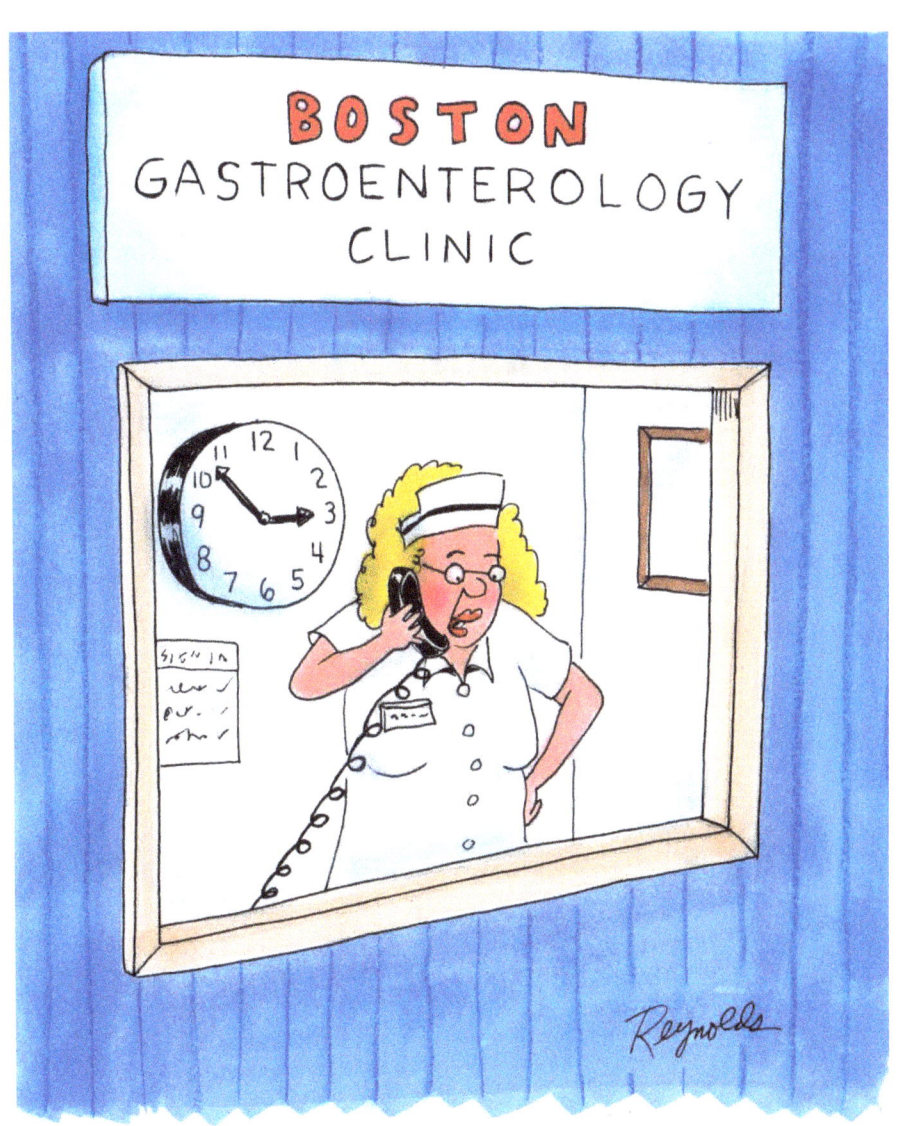

"No, I don't have an accent. I said your appointment was *too farty*."

Canaries were used for safety in coal mines, with its sudden death a warning of the presence of methane.

Cockroaches fart every fifteen minutes.

The average cow produces enough methane to power a one-hundred-watt light bulb for twenty-four hours.

The fart bubble of a blue whale is so large when it rises to the surface of the ocean it can envelope and asphyxiate both a horse and its rider.

Going up in an elevator in a high-rise building can cause an increase in farting, because intestinal gasses expand as the atmospheric pressure decreases with ascent.

The gastrointestinal tract is twenty-three feet long, about the vertical height of a two-story building.

The Fart Side: Blowing in the Wind!

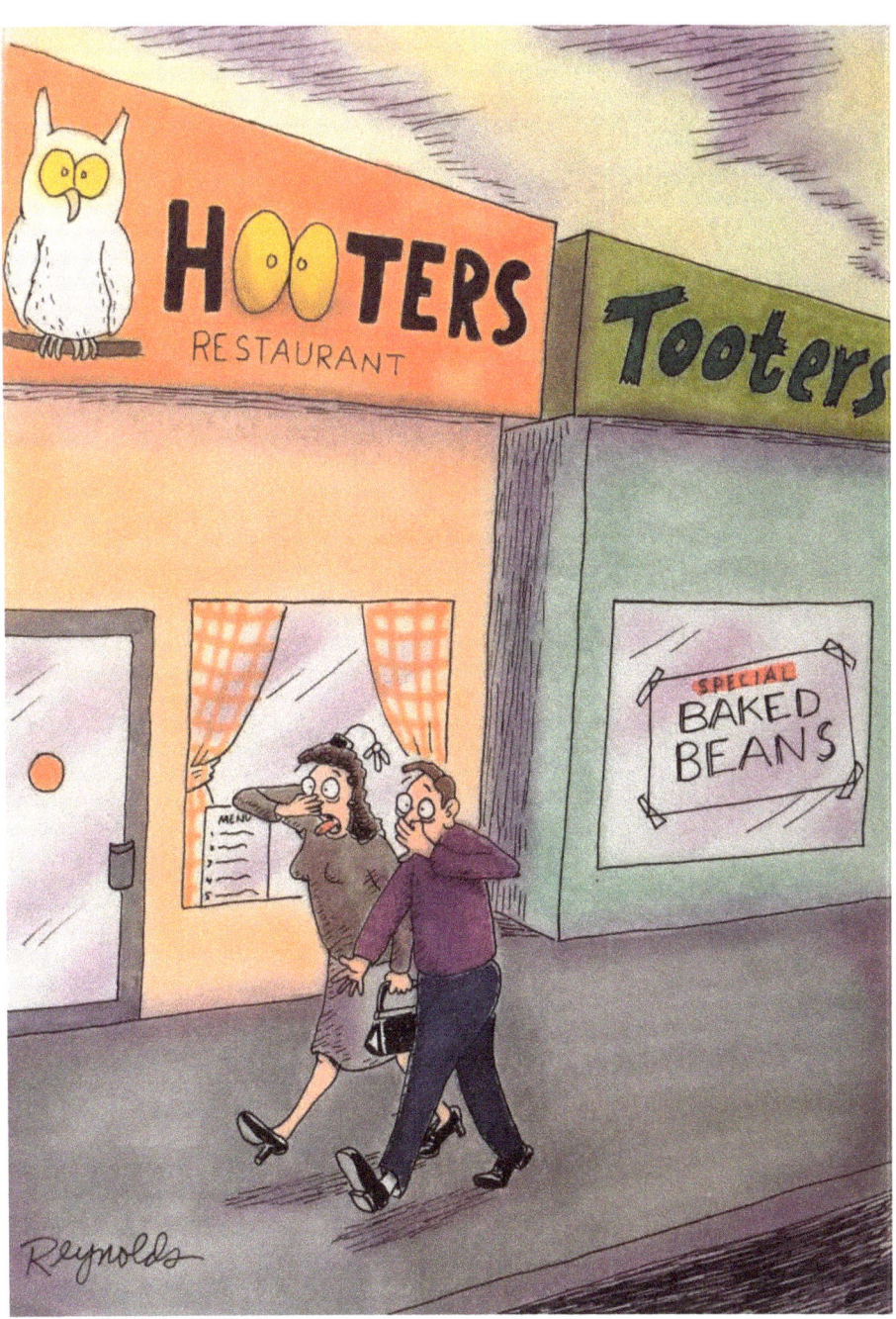

Petrified dinosaur poop, called a coprolite or coprolith, is a valuable find prized by paleontologists.

The dung beetle, which collects animal droppings as a food and nesting source, was considered sacred in Ancient Egypt.

The air we inhale contains less than one tenth of one percent carbon dioxide, the air we exhale has levels of carbon dioxide that is typically one hundred times as great.

The Pogonophoran Worm, the Jellyfish and the Coral and Sea Anemones cannot fart. This is a result of their anatomy, they do not have an anus.

A polysaccharide is a complex sugar, in which the molecules are composed of many glucose subunits arranged in a chain.

The Fart Side: Blowing in the Wind!

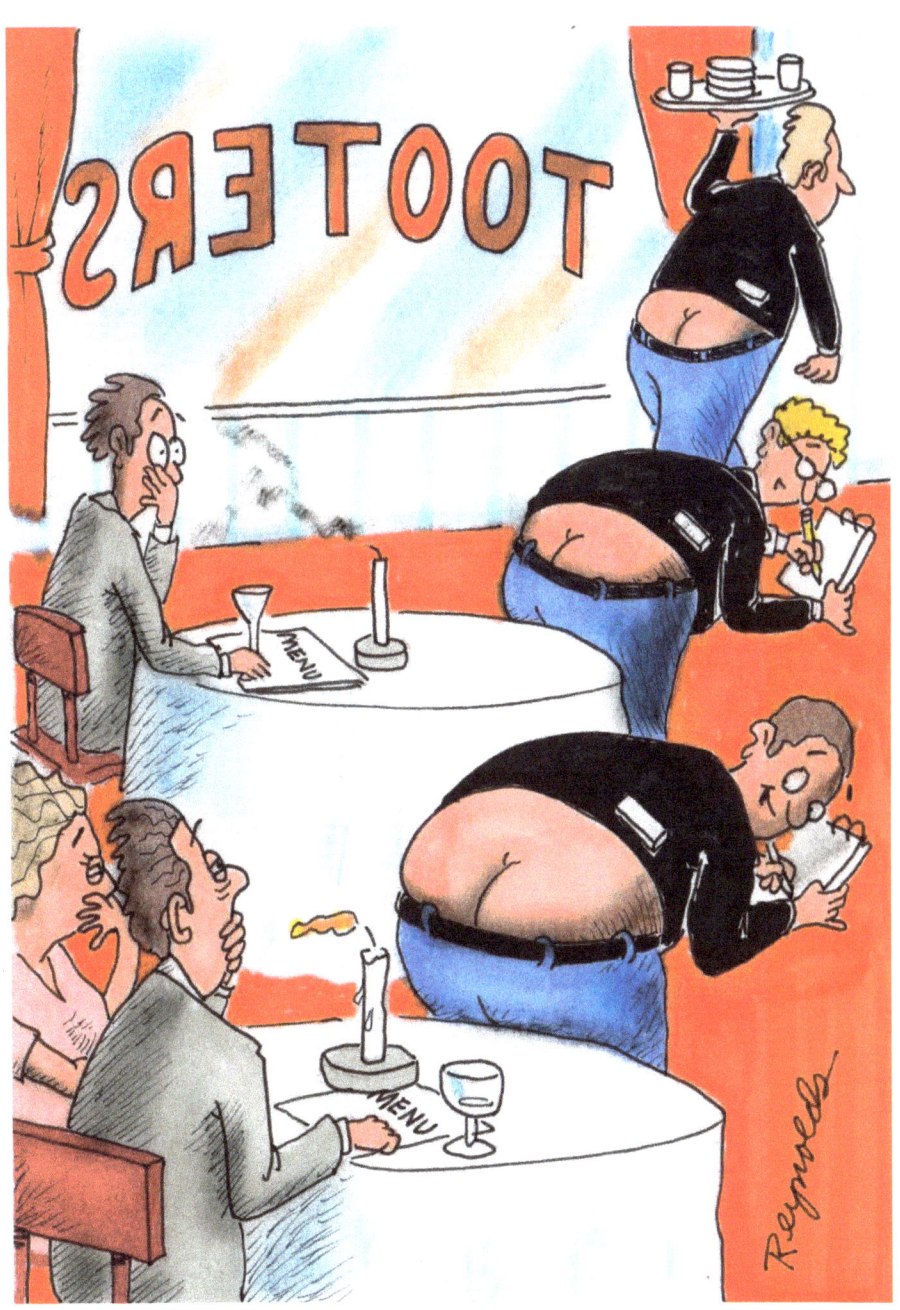

Although farts are usually invisible, they can be made readily visible by farting underwater.

The cause of the condition Celiac Sprue (Gluten Sensitive Enteropathy) was discovered because of a famine during World War Two. It occurs in one percent of the population.

Sea lions and other animals that eat large quantities of fish in their diet are reported to have the world's worst smelling farts.

Tropical beaches of white sand are created from the droppings of the parrotfish. They eat coral and the residue which they deposit, after it passes as poop, is considered sand.

Methane, which is odorless, is not produced by bacteria, but by other microbes known as Archaea.

The Fart Side: Blowing in the Wind!

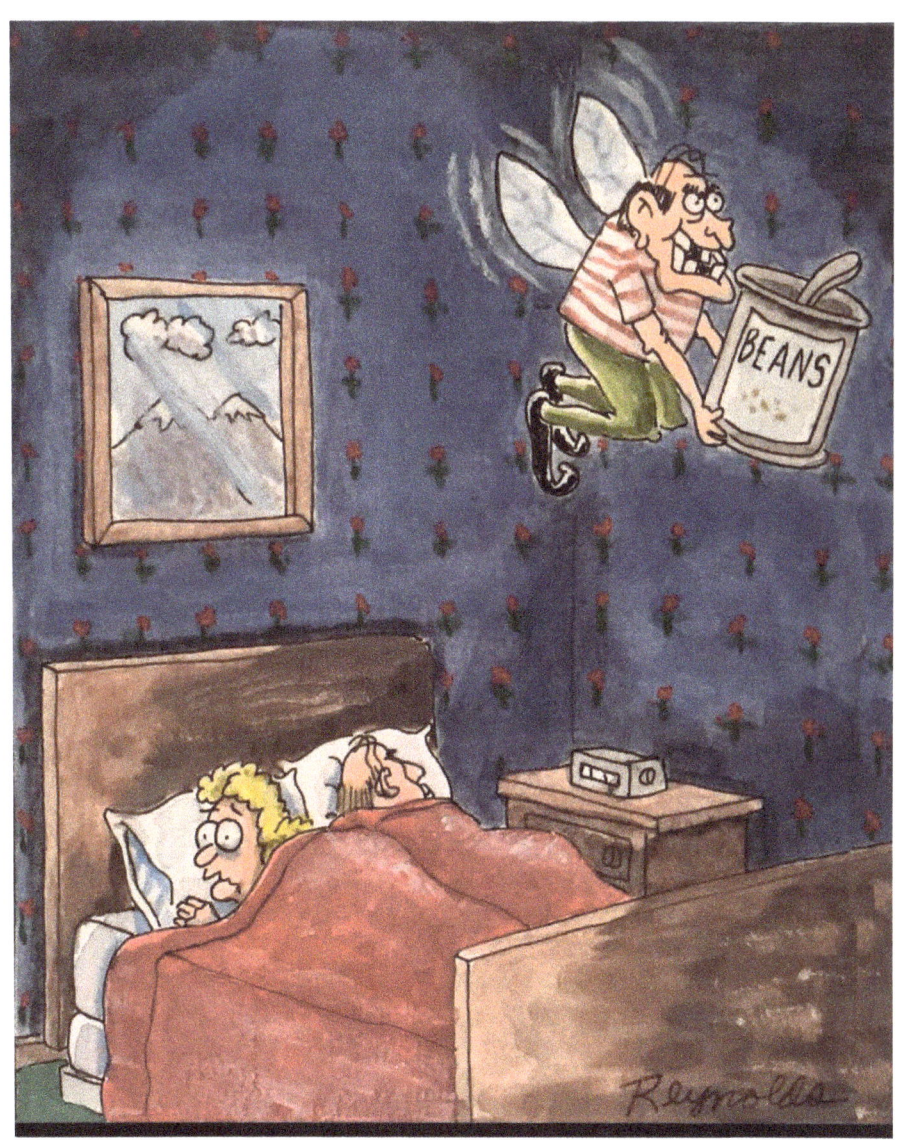

Late at night, much to Mrs. Murray's dismay, Mr. Murray would often receive a visit from the "Toot Fairy".

Manatees control their buoyancy by farting when they want to submerge, and letting intestinal gasses build up when they want to float.

The Fitzroy River Turtle of Australia has the unique ability to also be able to breathe through its cloaca / anus.

A carminative is a preparation or herb that promotes the elimination of gas from the gastrointestinal tract. Many carminatives have been shown to work by releasing air swallowed (aerophagia) as a burp.

There are on average one hundred times more bacterial contaminants on restaurant menus than on restaurant toilet seats.

The term gut refers to the digestive tract, also known as the alimentary canal or gastrointestinal tract.

The Fart Side: Blowing in the Wind!

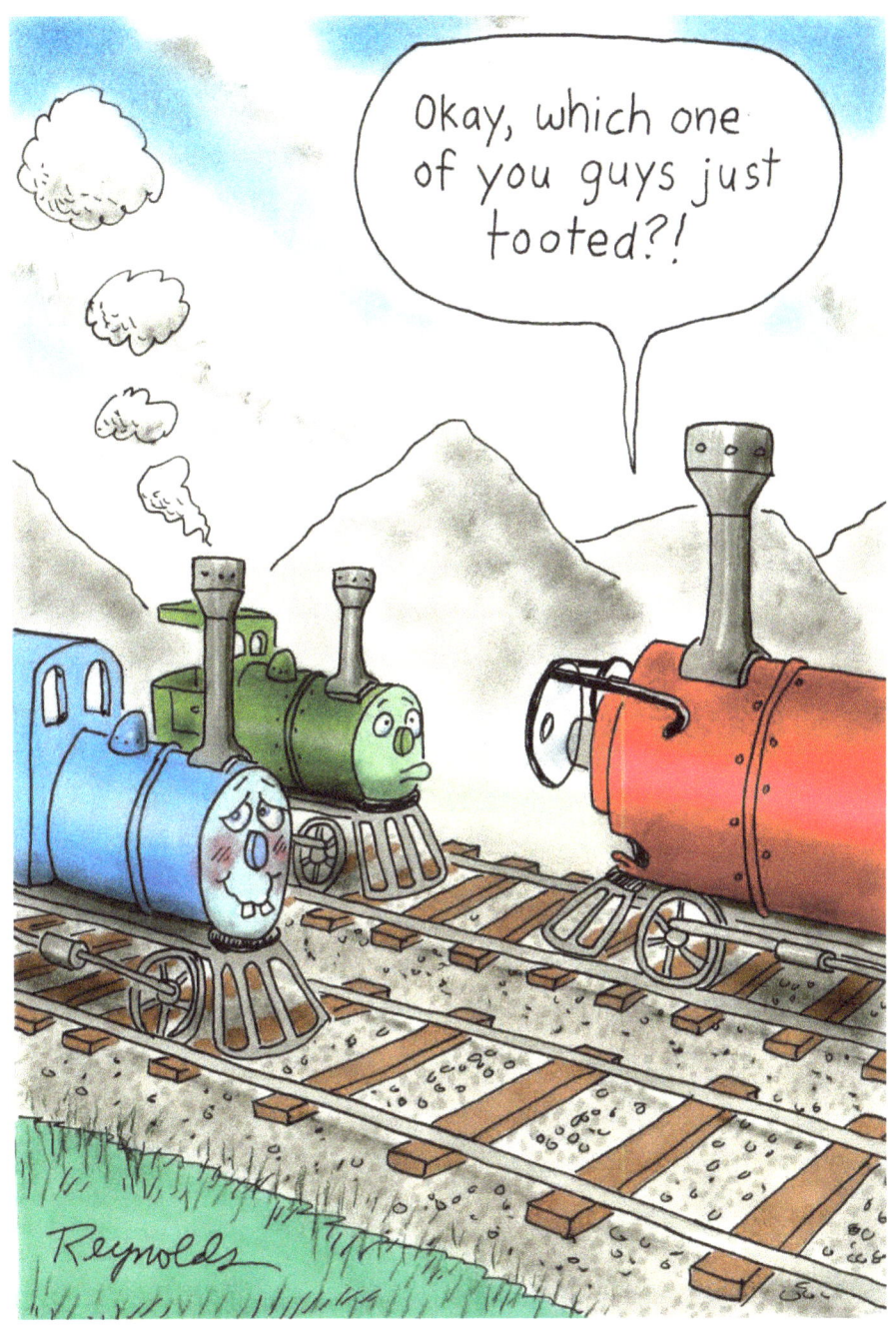

In Western culture, the most common product that people see and use for its carminative property is mint. It relaxes the lower esophageal sphincter to encourage eructation. It can also contribute to reflux and heartburn.

Chocolate can have a similar effect, so it is often offered in combination as an after-dinner chocolate mint.

Indian and Asian restaurants may offer other more traditional carminative herbs and seeds, usually found on the counter by the exit.

Women burp more during pregnancy because of the effect of hormones, as well as the increased abdominal pressure from the growing fetus.

The term organic is applied to compounds that contain the chemical elements of carbon and hydrogen.

The Fart Side: Blowing in the Wind!

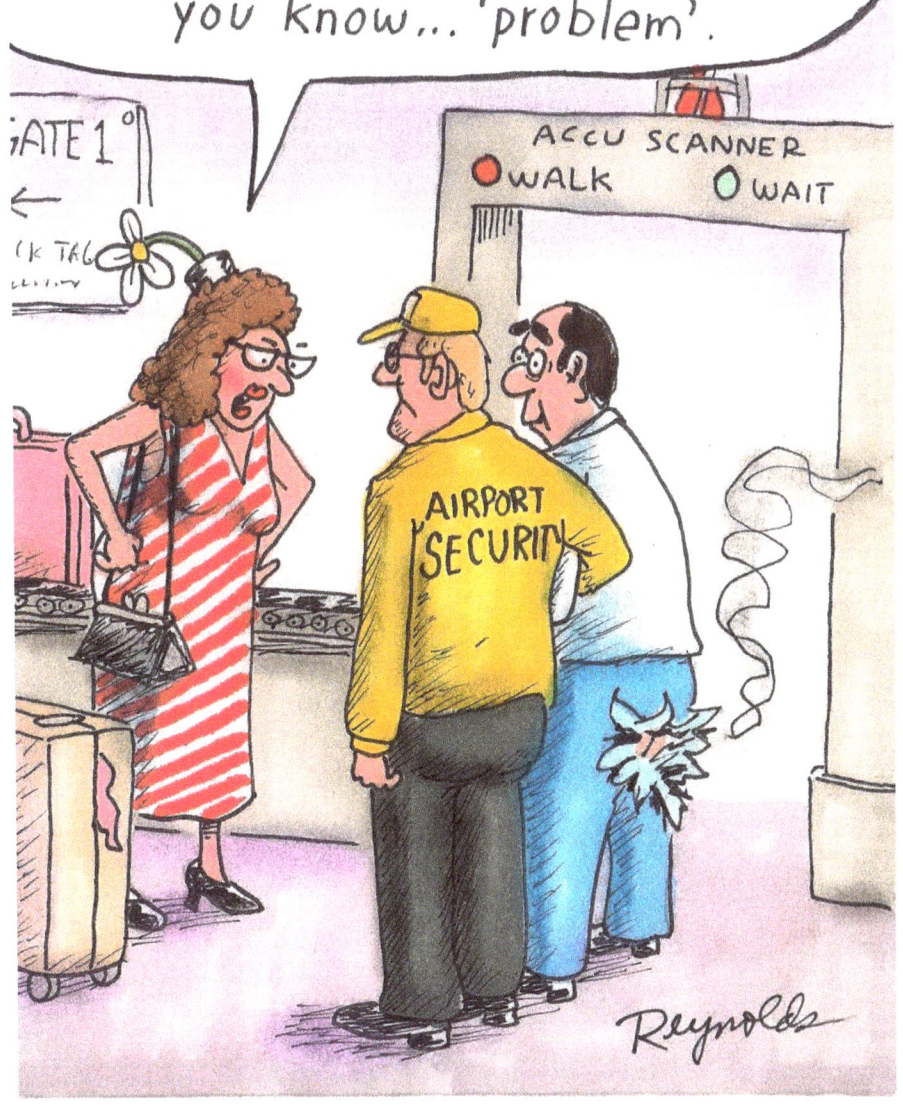

The World Burping Federation holds an annual championship. The *Guinness Book of World Records* has a listing for the loudest burp on record. The record holder is Paul Hunn whose burp achieved a measurement of 109.9 decibels, equivalent to a car horn.

The world record for the longest burp is 18.1 seconds, held by Tim Janus. To achieve this record, he consumed approximately two gallons of Diet Coke and Mountain Dew.

Without stomach acid, digestion can still take place.

Raw Lima beans contain cyanide and can cause illness and death if consumed in excess.

An organ is a group of specialized cells and tissues organized into a structure, that performs a specific function.

The Fart Side: Blowing in the Wind!

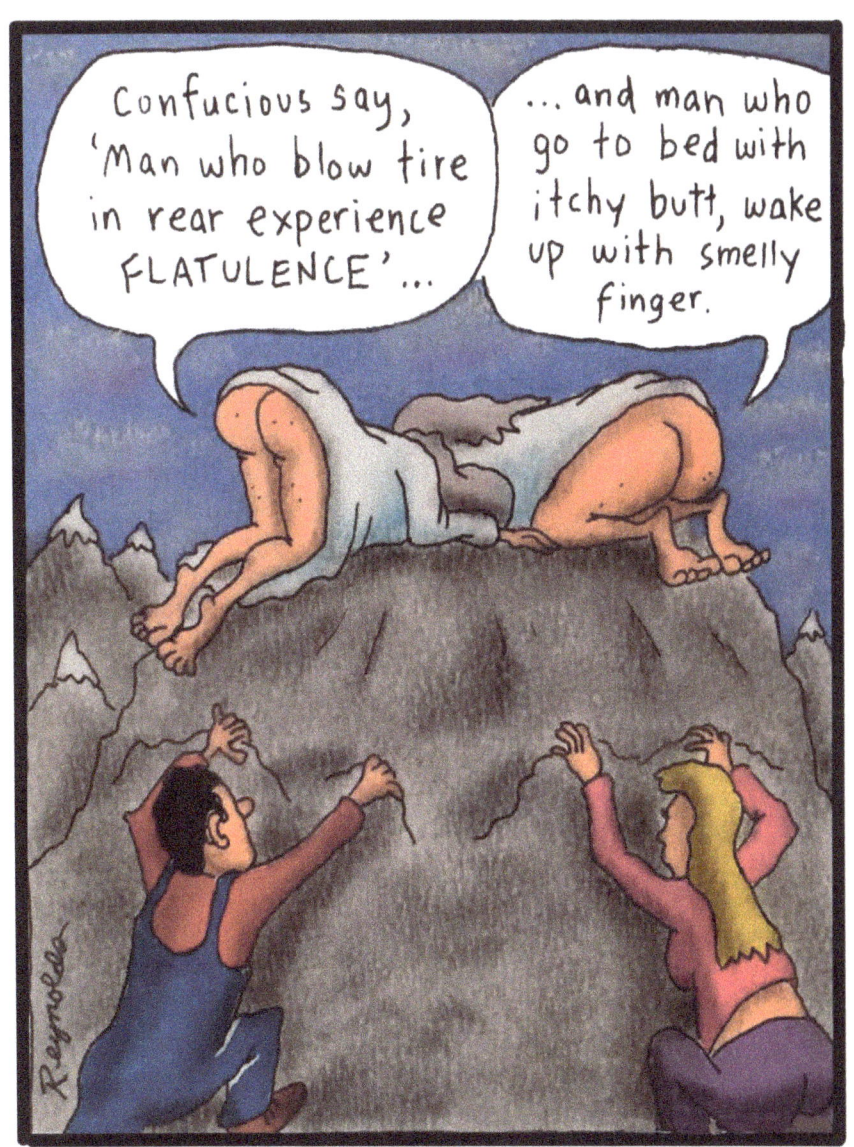

With the average human swallowing over two thousand times per day, about ten liters of air are ingested every single day. That is about eight liters of poorly absorbed nitrogen that has been taken in, and now needs to get out. The most direct exit, the shortest distance to travel, and the fastest way to get relief, is to burp or belch.

That is more gas in the digestive tract than the most frequent and dedicated burpers and belchers can release through eructation. The nitrogen contributes to bloating, before it eventually makes its way out of the other end of the intestinal tract as a fart. Air swallowing (aerophagia) is a major contributor to farting.

Beets can cause the stool to appear blood red in color, and discolor toilet bowl water to look like blood.

The Fart Side: Blowing in the Wind!

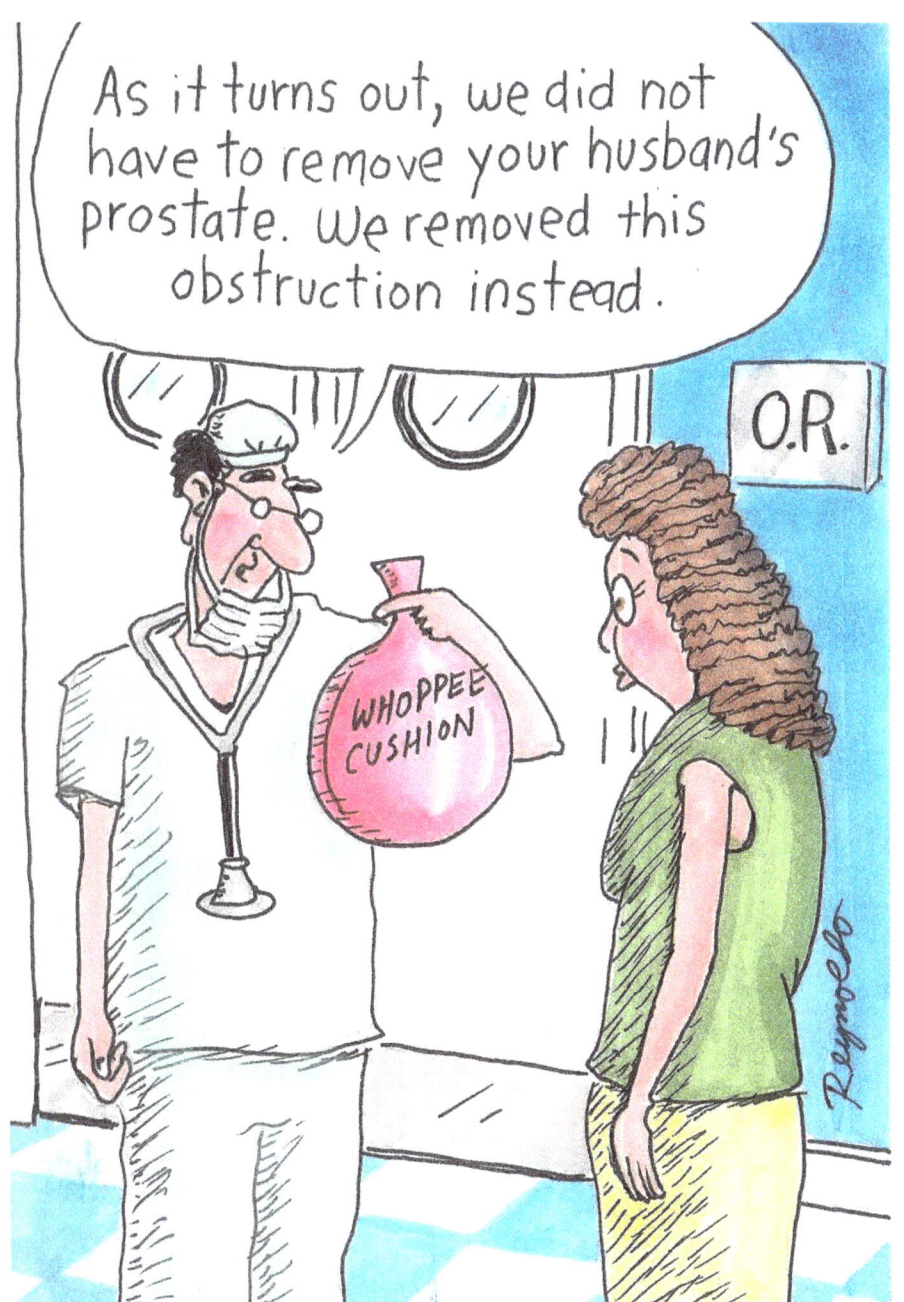

A hidden source of swallowed air is the air content present within many foods. Fruits contain a large amount of air. If you compress an apple, and add the volume of the juice and the pressed fruit together, you will find that it was only sixty percent of the volume of the original fruit, forty percent was air.

Ice cream contains a lot of air, up to fifty percent of its volume. An easy way to demonstrate this is take a full container of ice cream you bought at the store, and let it melt. As it melts the air trapped inside the ice cream is released, and you will discover that the container of ice cream was nearly half full of air.

Internal bleeding in the digestive tract, or ingesting blood, may produce a black tar-like stool known as melena. Iron, bismuth, and black licorice can give stool a black color, not melena.

The Fart Side: Blowing in the Wind!

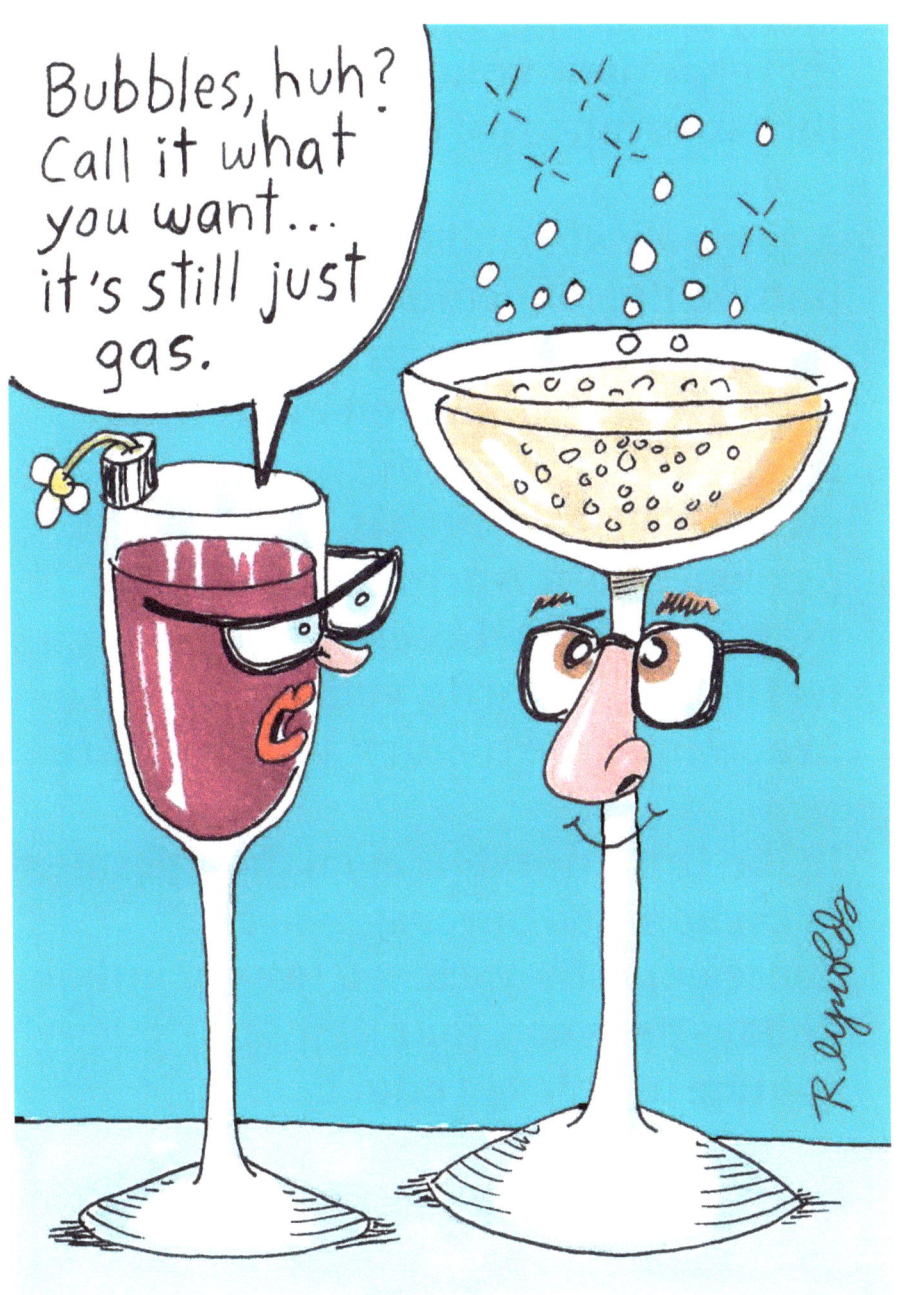

Many foods are whipped with air to increase their volume, which adds to the smoothness of the product.

Adding air also contributes to the bottom line of profitability for the manufacturer. Most products are sold for a higher price when the volume is increased. For the consumer, the swallowed air, which is nearly eighty percent non-absorbable nitrogen, must be released as either a burp or a fart. In other words, you are paying a premium price to burp and fart more.

In the United States, even though sales of carbonated beverages are decreasing, they exceed twenty billion dollars per year, four times the sales volume of dairy products.

Calcium containing antacids can cause a rebound increase in gastric acid secretion.

The Fart Side: Blowing in the Wind!

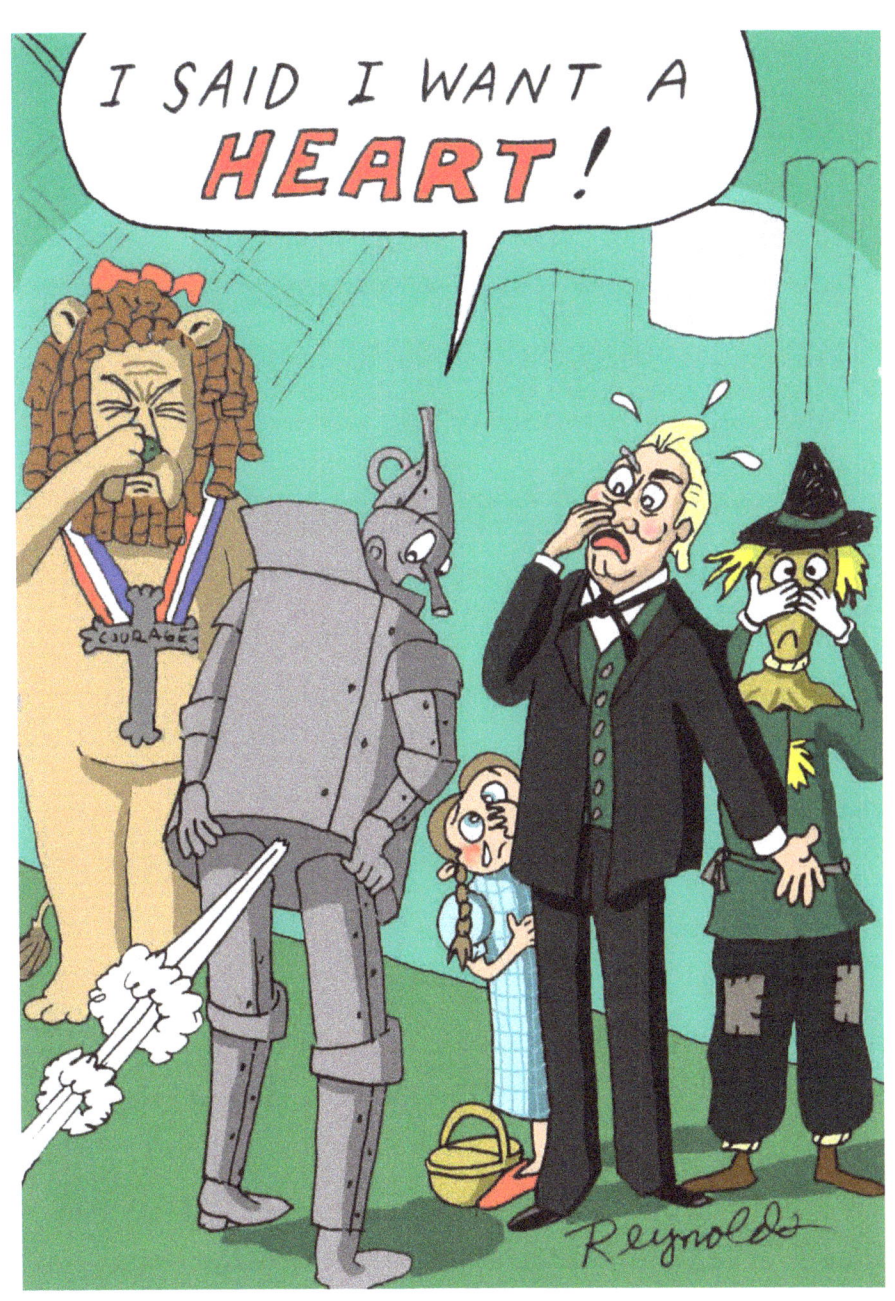

With every single swallow about five milliliters, or one teaspoonful, of air is swallowed. This occurs whether you are eating, drinking, or just resting between meals. You swallow approximately every thirty seconds while awake, and about every five minutes while asleep.

Swallowing of a liquid is more complex than the swallowing of a solid.

The average person swallows about two thousand times a day, but many swallow much more than that.

Air is seventy-eight percent nitrogen, which is a poorly absorbed gas. If it is not released in a burp, it will lead to bloating, distension, and farting.

Alka-Seltzer and Pepto-Bismol contain aspirin derivatives known as salicylates.

The Fart Side: Blowing in the Wind!

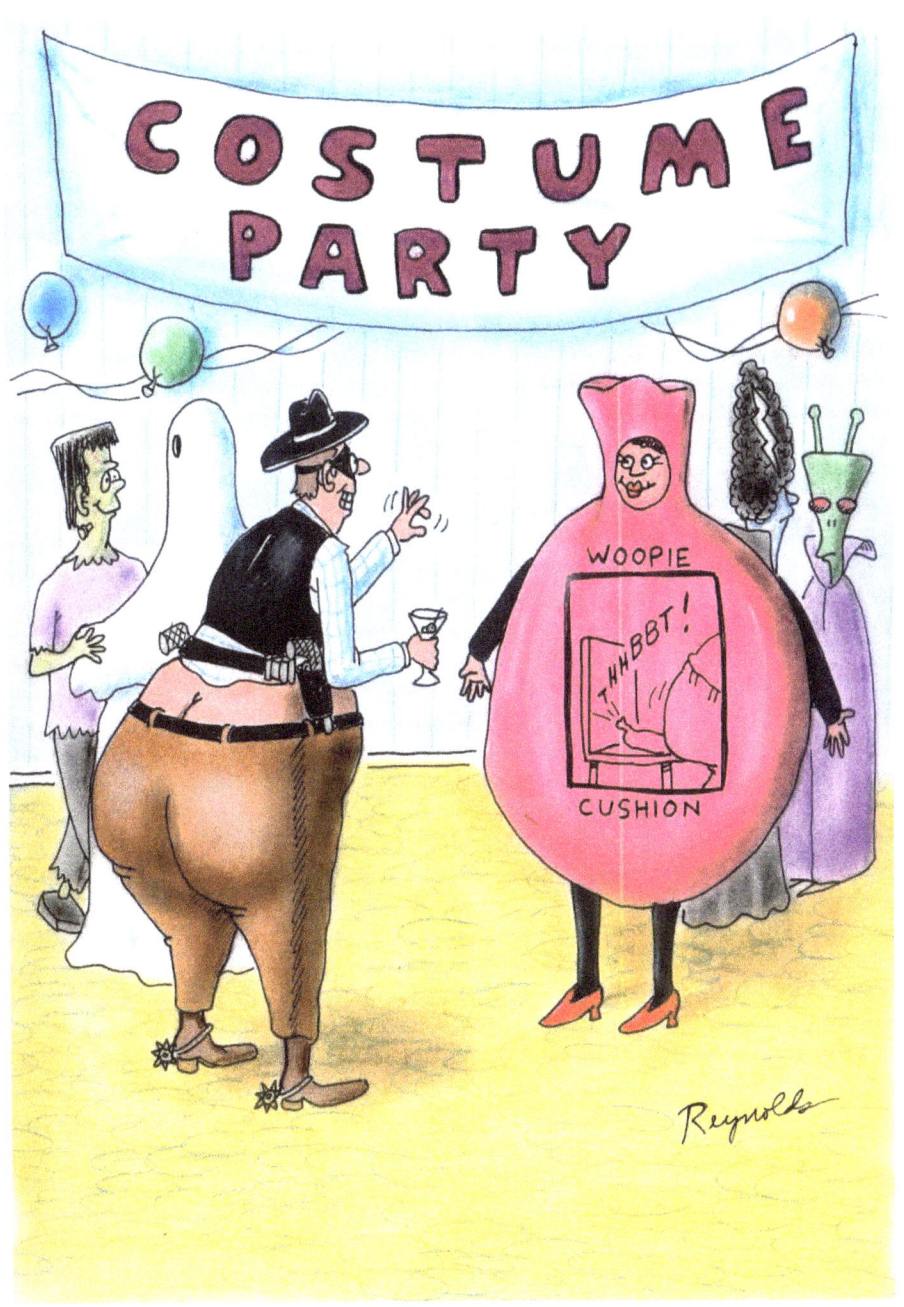

The only large mammal that is unable to burp is the horse. Unlike cattle which are ruminants with several stomachs, horses have only one stomach. The valve into the stomach opens only one way, so horses cannot regurgitate, burp, belch, or vomit.

Most people burp between six and twenty times a day.

Although it is not recommended, you can swallow while standing on your head, since the strength of peristalsis can overcome the force of gravity.

Human digestion does not remove all nutrient value from the food ingested, so the waste product of feces has remaining nutritional value.

Sphincter is a general term for a muscle that surrounds, and can control the size of, a bodily opening.

The Fart Side: Blowing in the Wind!

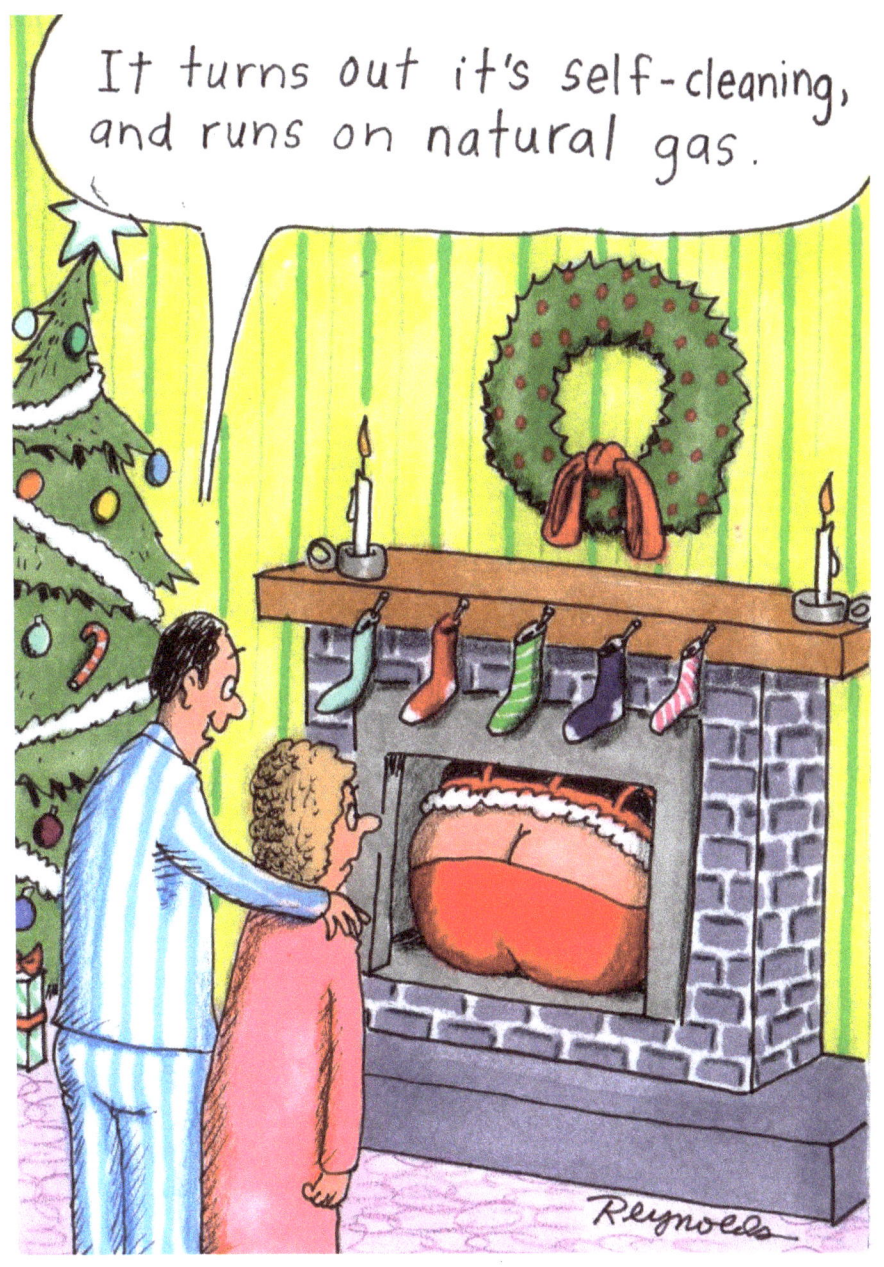

The official medical term for burping is eructation.

The holes in Swiss cheese arise from microbial gas production.

Every year cows in the U.S.A. burp about fifty million tons of methane gas into the atmosphere.

The burps of ten cows could heat a small house for a year.

Rats, rabbits, guinea pigs, chickens, and horses can't vomit or burp.

A hiccup is caused by the involuntary contraction of the diaphragm.

Borborygmus is the name given to audible stomach growls and sounds.

Most people pass more than ten farts per day.

The Fart Side: Blowing in the Wind!

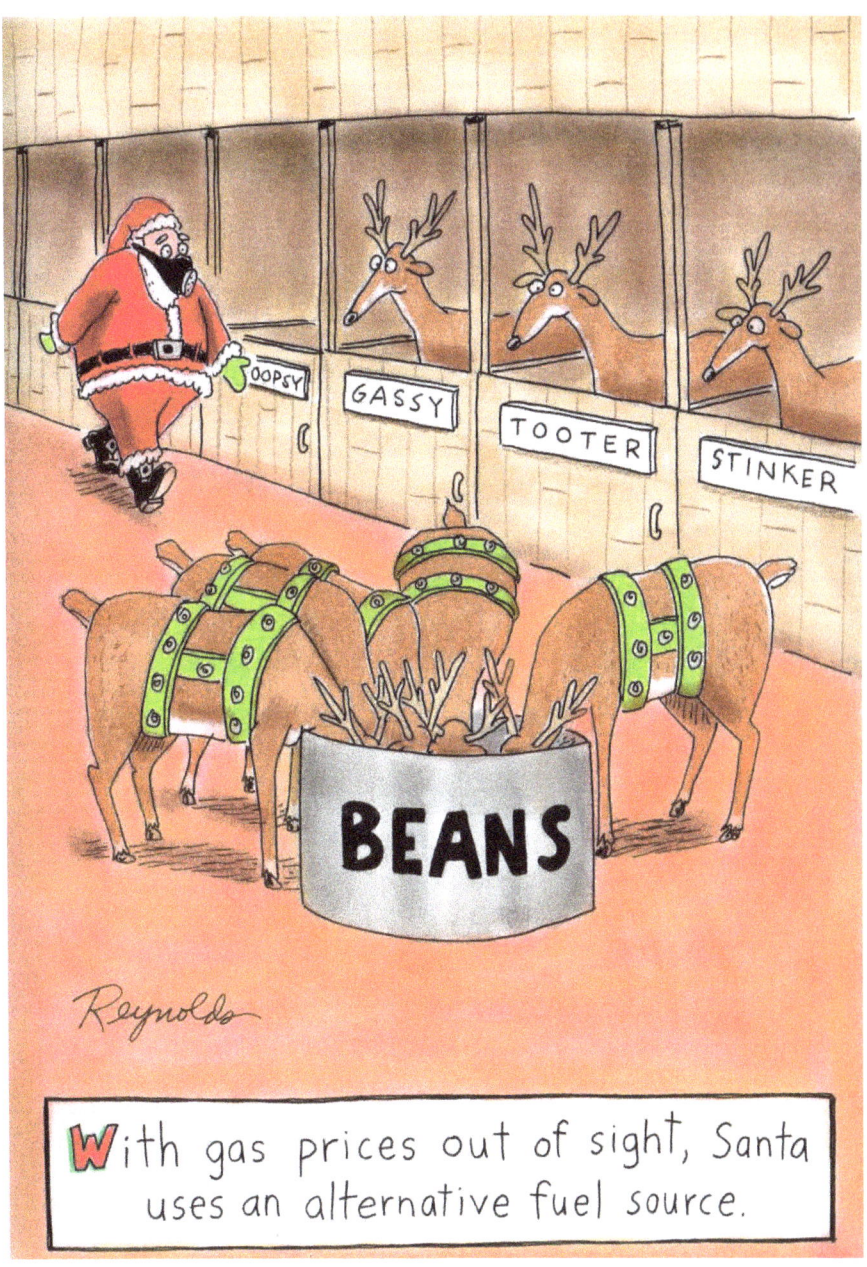

Toilet paper must be at least ten sheets thick to prevent fecal contamination of the hands with wiping.

Poor fitting dentures can contribute to intestinal gas.

Drinking a cold carbonated beverage will release greater volumes of gas than drinking the same type and quantity of beverage served at room temperature.

Drinking the same quantity of a carbonated beverage, at the same temperature, will release more gas if consumed in Denver than in Miami, due to the difference in atmospheric pressure and altitude.

Peptic ulcers are painful sores on the lining of the esophagus, stomach or small intestine, and affect nearly fifty million Americans each year.

The Fart Side: Blowing in the Wind!

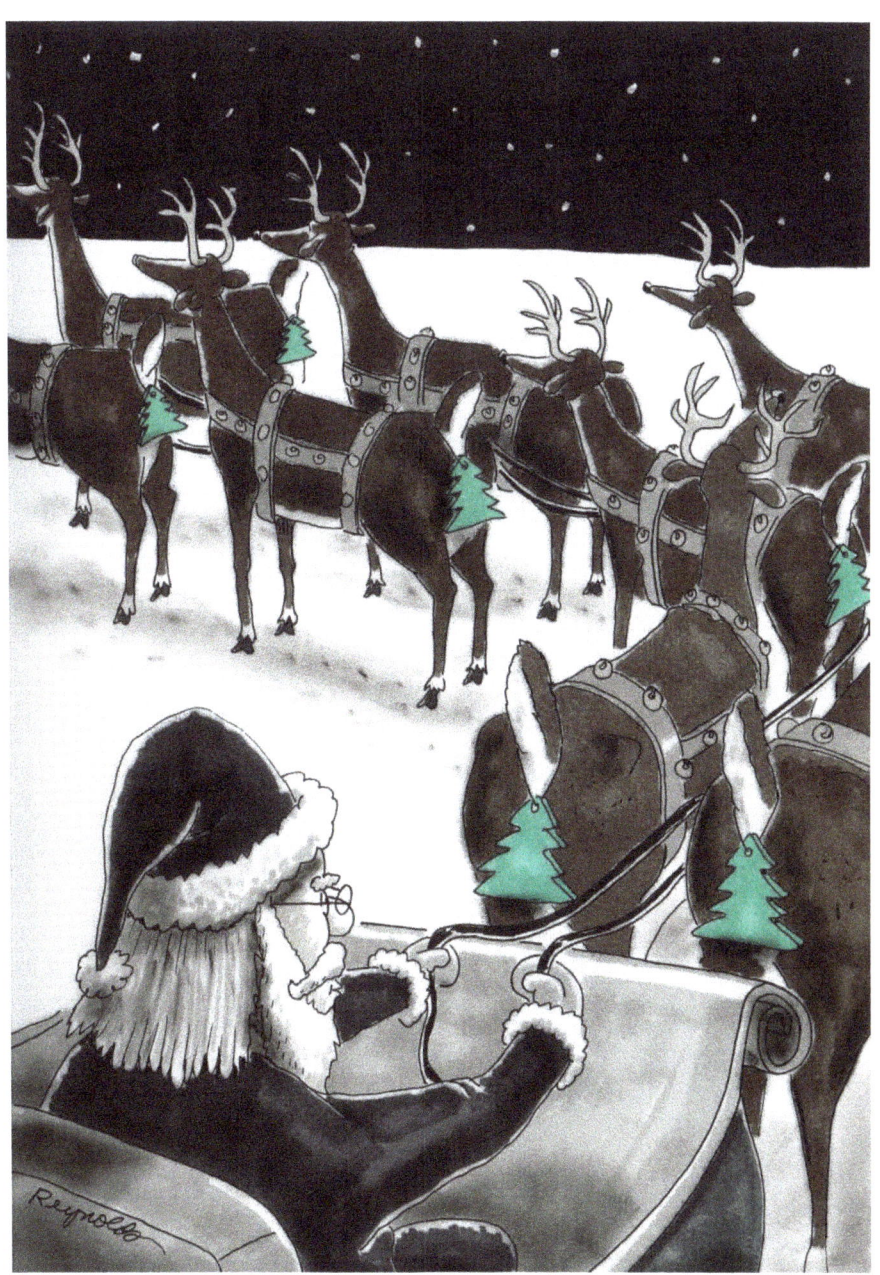

Carbonated beverages outsell dairy products by a ratio of four to one in the United States.

Bloodhounds, which have the keenest sense of smell of any dogs, have noses up to one-hundred-million times more sensitive than a human's. Put into terms of a visual acuity analogy, it is as if the text on the page of this book could be read at two thousand miles.

Kellogg's Corn Flakes was developed by a physician, John Harvey Kellogg, specifically to address bowel health.

Graham Crackers were developed by a minister as a food with high fiber and roughage that was thought to aid in the suppression of masturbation.

Rapid weight loss is a risk factor for the development of gallstones.

The Fart Side: Blowing in the Wind!

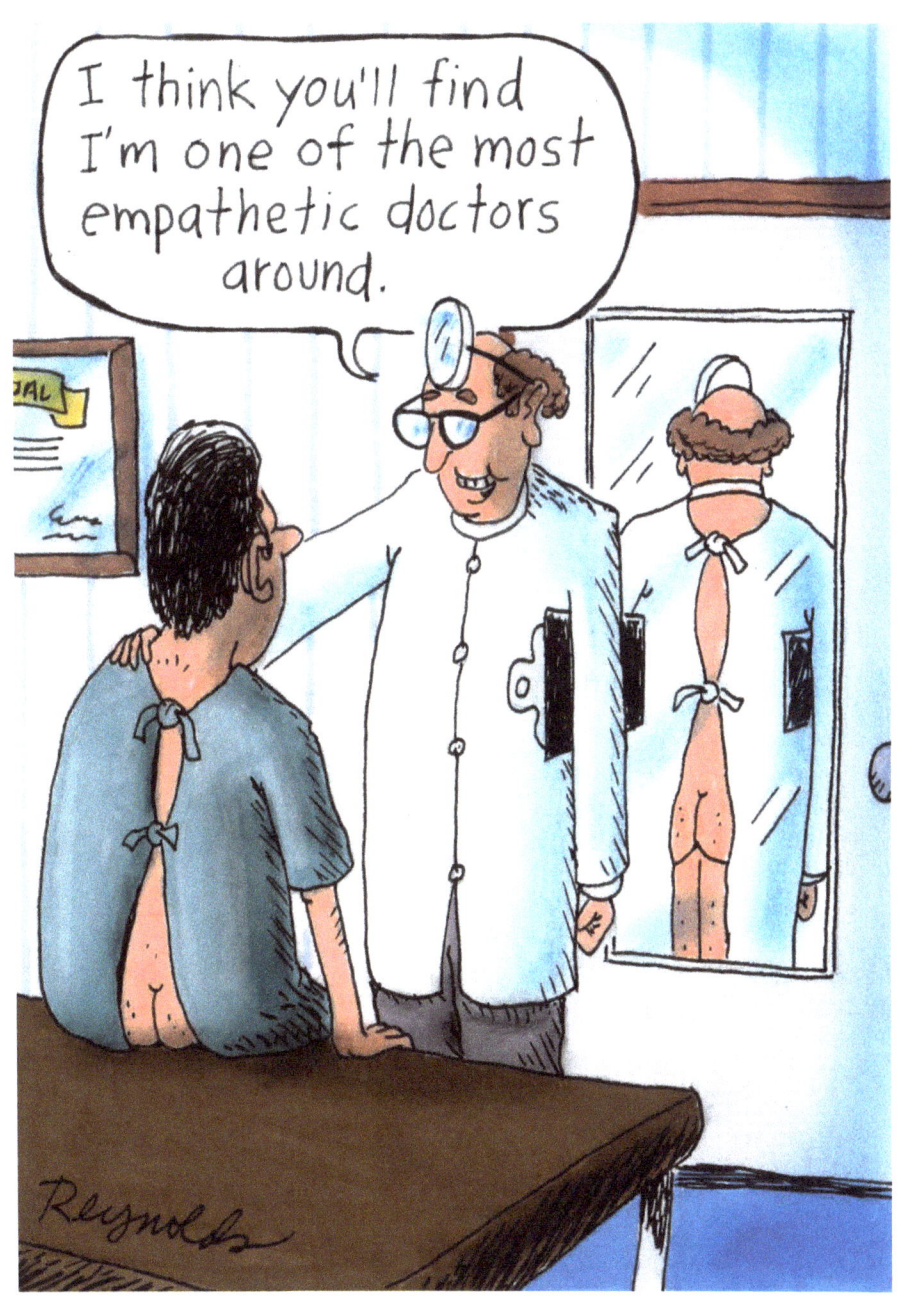

Gut bacteria produce vitamin K and the B vitamins.

Bacteria in feces produce sulfur- or nitrogen-rich compounds such as indole, skatole, and mercaptans, and the inorganic gas hydrogen sulfide. These give stool and farts their characteristic fecal odor.

On occasion people may harbor a yeast that converts plant sugars into alcohol, which is then absorbed and can lead to intoxication, even without drinking an alcoholic beverage.

Humans produce on average one to two liters (quarts) of saliva per day.

The medical term for swallowing is deglutition.

Zinc is important for the perception of taste & texture of food.

The Fart Side: Blowing in the Wind!

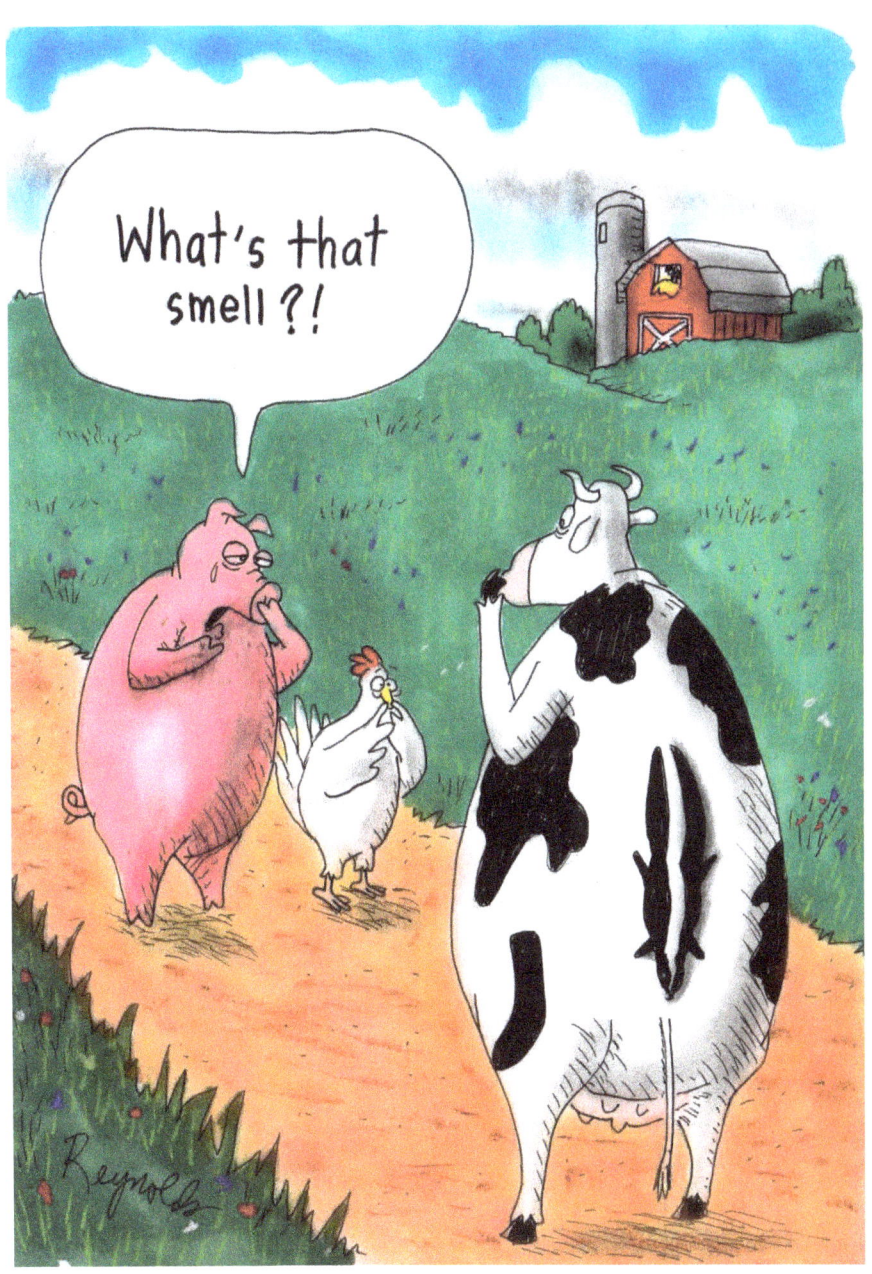

The average person goes to the toilet 2,500 times per year, and spends a total of three years of their lifetime sitting on the toilet.

For those musically inclined, most toilets flush in the key of E flat.

Sugar cane was processed in India over two thousand five hundred years ago, and was called khanda. This is the original word from which the English word candy is derived.

In many parts of the world, popular and religious custom dictate that only the left hand be used for wiping after a bowel movement. The right hand is reserved for food handling and social interactions. This is believed to be the origin of the right-hand shake as a greeting, since the left hand was considered unclean.

The Fart Side: Blowing in the Wind!

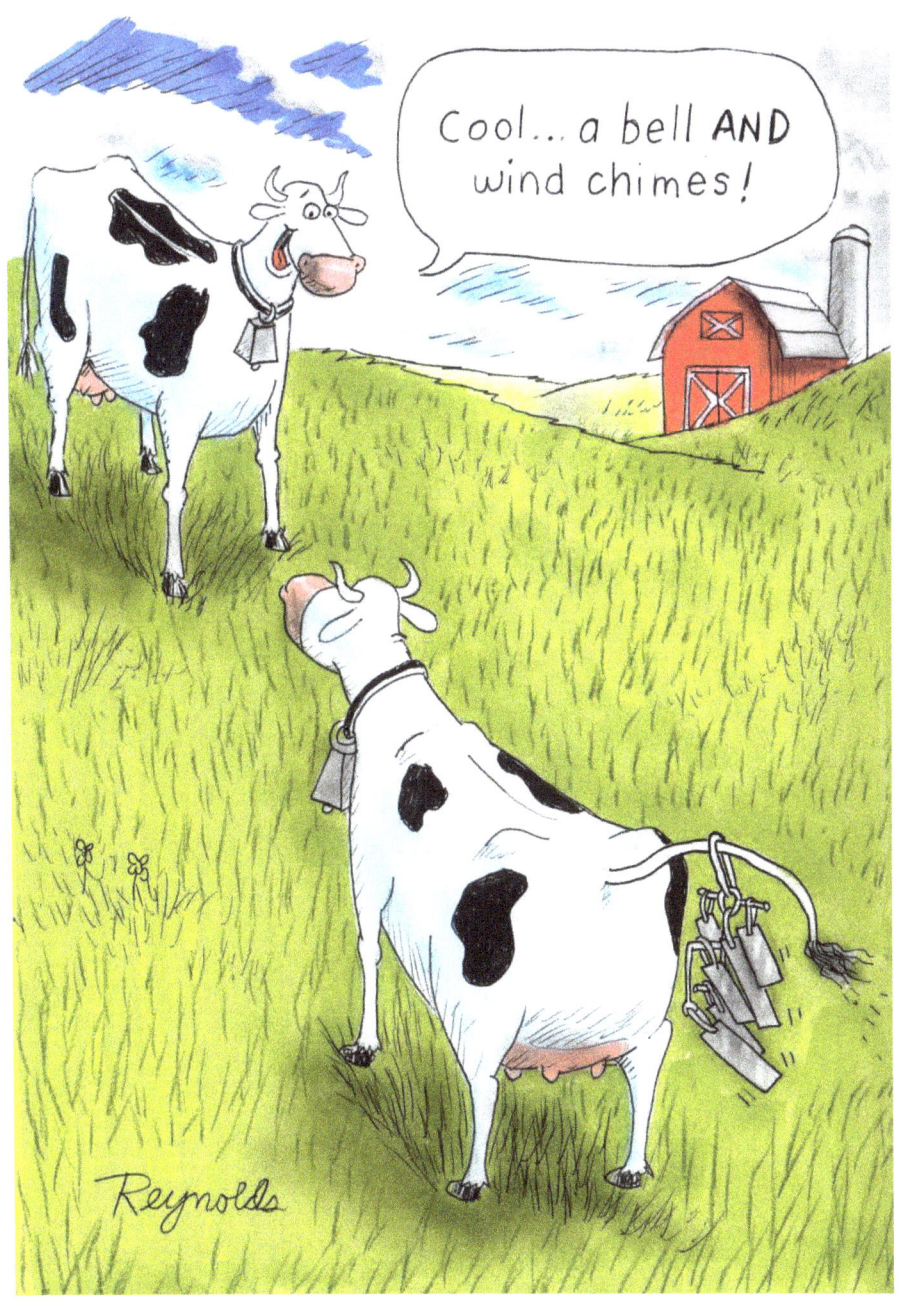

The flushing of a toilet will aerosolize fecal microbes that would cover a room, with dimensions of twenty feet by twenty feet, in a matter of seconds.

The use of human feces as a fertilizer, known as night soil, is common in many parts of the world.

In Japan, the fecal waste of rich people was more expensive as night soil. This was because it was thought to have greater nutritional value, since the wealthy were presumed to have a better diet.

Toilet paper is very porous and allows fecal contamination of the hands of most people with wiping. This is why toilet paper is inferior to a water bidet for anal hygiene.

Your body coordinates quadrillions of chemical reactions per second.

The Fart Side: Blowing in the Wind!

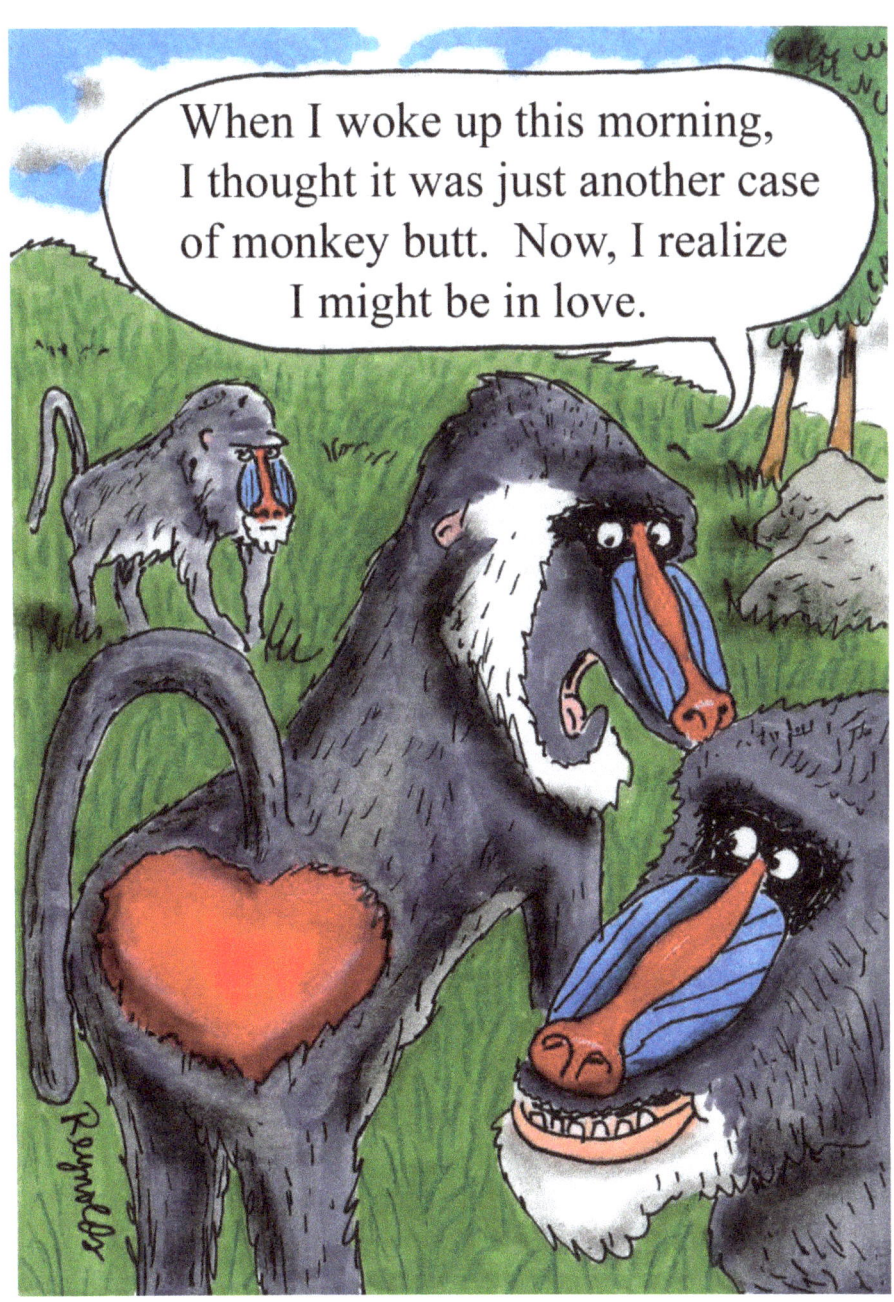

Hemorrhoids are part of normal human anatomy, and have an important function in maintaining fecal continence.

Toilet flush handles have over four hundred times as many fecal bacterial contaminants as the toilet seat.

More than twenty-five billion rolls of toilet paper are sold every year in the U.S.

Specially designed toilets in the space shuttle and International Space Station have seat restraints so that astronauts do not lift off the toilet seat, because a fart released in weightlessness can act as a propulsive force.

The largest of the salivary glands are the parotid glands, which can become swollen with the viral condition called mumps.

The Fart Side: Blowing in the Wind!

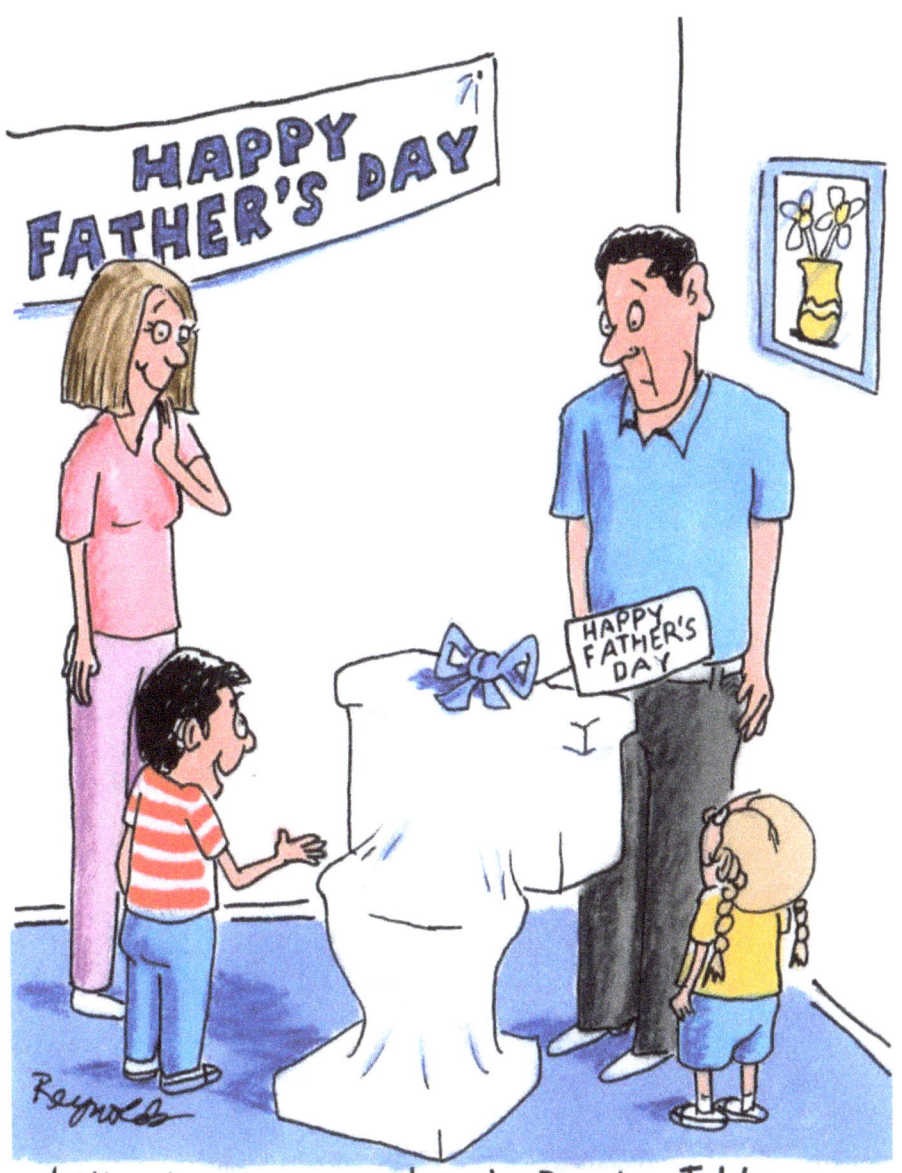

The pair of salivary glands underneath the jaw are the submandibular glands, and produce both serous fluid and mucus. Another pair of salivary glands are the sublingual glands located underneath the tongue. Their secretion is mainly mucous with a small percentage of saliva.

Over half the population over the age of fifty have a hiatal hernia that can lead to indigestion, heartburn, and gastroesophageal reflux.

Passengers in an elevator in a high-rise building are more likely to fart going up than going down.

Rapid changes in atmospheric pressure can occur with scuba diving, as well as aerospace travel. This can result in intestinal gas distention, and on rare occasions, barotrauma leading to perforation, peritonitis, and death.

The Fart Side: Blowing in the Wind!

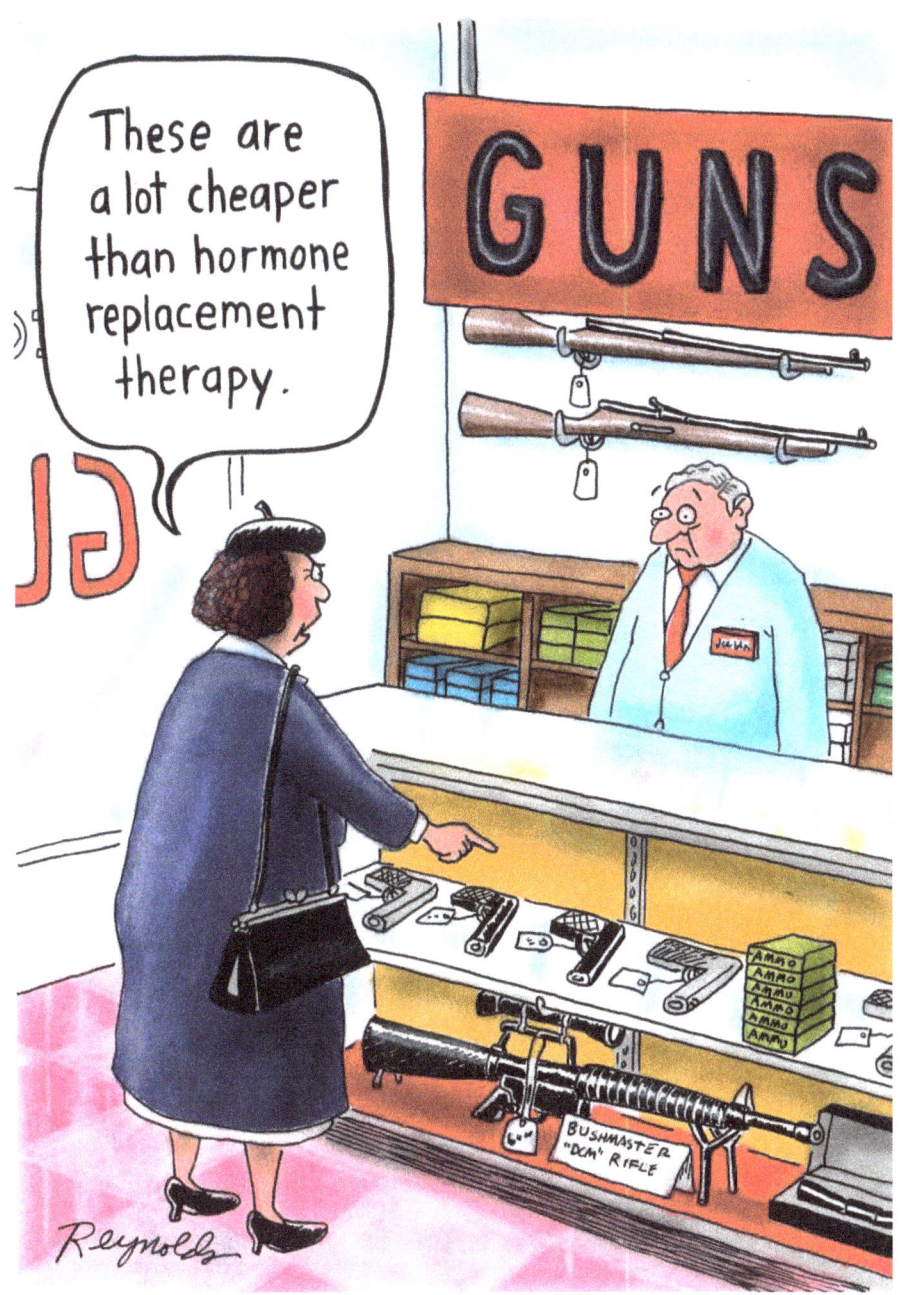

Cranial Nerve X (Ten), the vagus nerve, travels from the brain to the lungs, heart, gut, and other internal organs. The word is derived from the Latin 'vagus' which means wanderer, since it wanders anatomically through so many organs.

The oxygen content of the air in the passenger compartment of a traveling airplane is substantially lower than the atmosphere at ground level.

According to the laws of physics, developing a fever will lead to the volume expansion of pockets of intestinal gas.

The microbes that reside in the gut are known as the gut microbiome.

The saliva from the parotid glands are predominantly watery serous secretion.

The Fart Side: Blowing in the Wind!

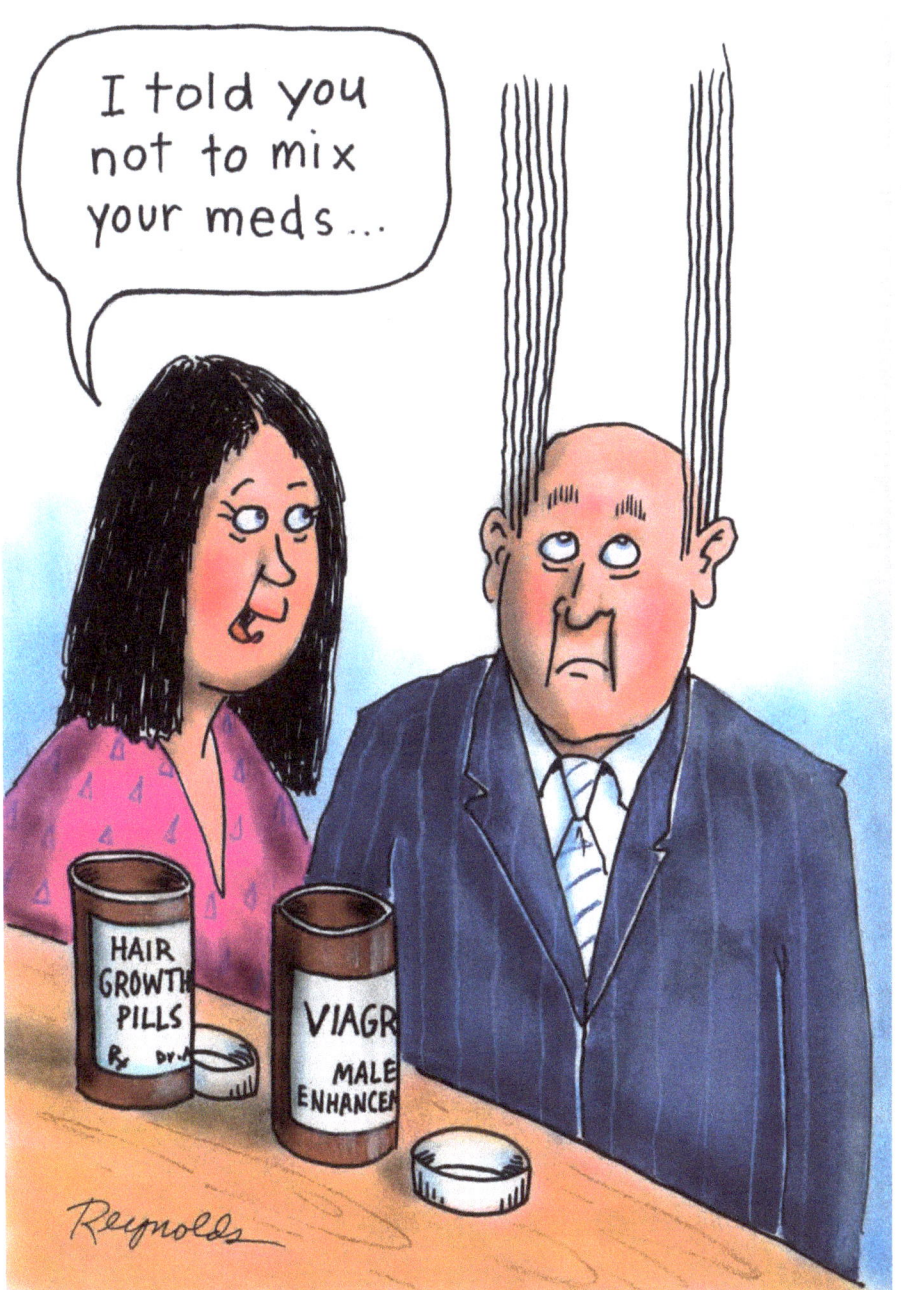

Hydrogen is the lightest and most abundant element, comprising ninety percent of all atoms, and seventy-five percent of all matter in the visible universe.

The term mammal is derived from the medical name for breasts, mammary glands. Feeding their young milk is one of the characteristics of the species.

Lactose is a common additive to foods and pharmaceutical products as a filler, and may trigger symptoms in those who are lactose intolerant, especially since it is often not clearly labeled as an ingredient.

Hypolactasia is the term for lactose intolerance and lactase deficiency.

The serous fluid is produced in the salivary glands contain lingual lipase, which helps to digest fats.

The Fart Side: Blowing in the Wind!

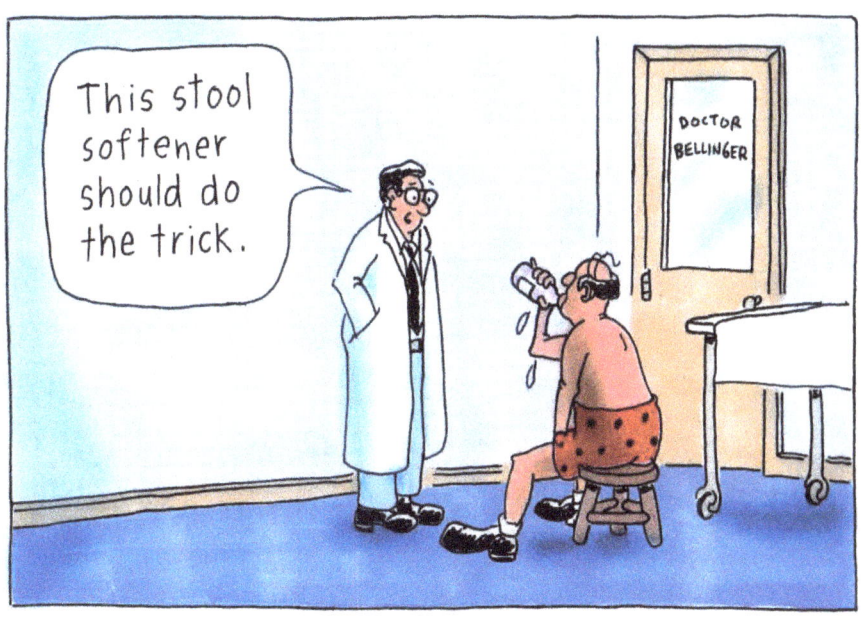

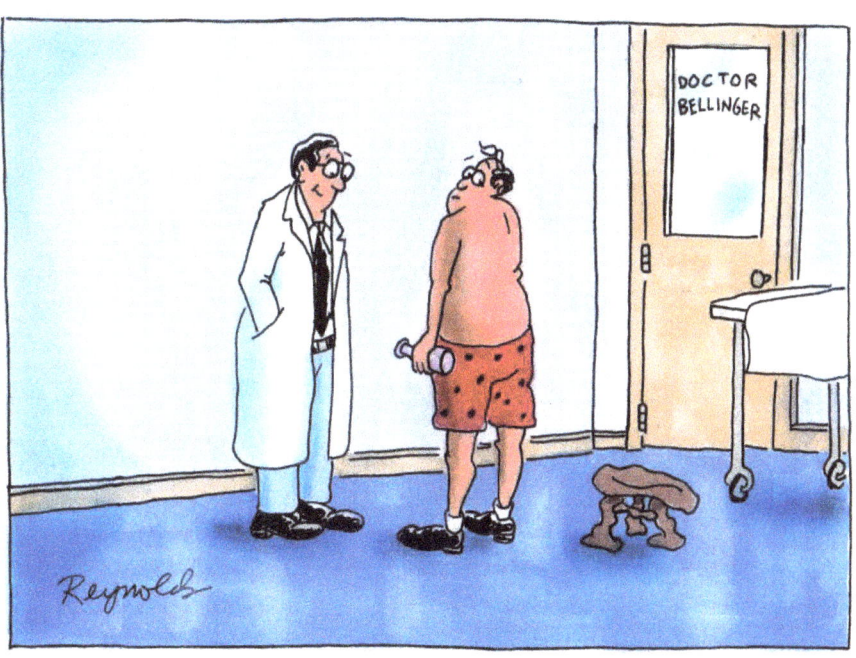

Seventy-five percent of African-American, Jewish, Native American, and Mexican American populations are lactose intolerant.

A high fat meal can increase intestinal gas by slowing down gut motility and allowing more microbial fermentation.

It takes exercise consuming three thousand five hundred calories of energy, to burn off one pound of body fat.

Some bacteria populations double every ten minutes, so that one bacterium can become four trillion in just seven hours. Overwhelming infections can kill humans in just a matter of hours from exposure.

Amylase is found in saliva and begins the digestive process of carbohydrates, breaking starches into simple sugars.

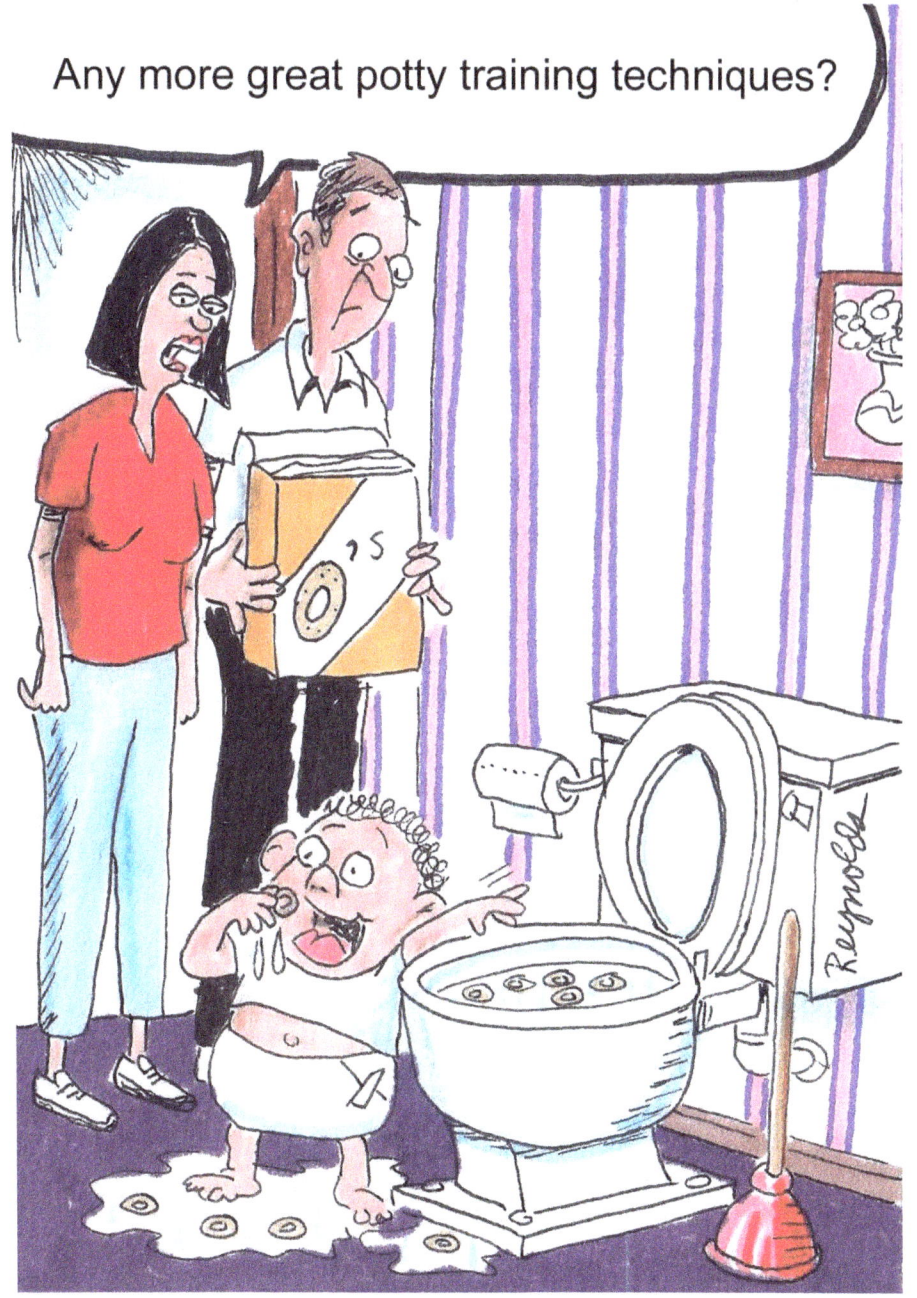

Even though they are dairy products, hard cheeses and yogurt often have low lactose content.

The production of sauerkraut, cheese, soy sauce, pickles, wine, yogurt, vinegar, breads, and cake could not occur without microbial activity.

Only a small percent of the species of microbes on earth have been identified, with millions of species remaining undiscovered.

Extremophile organisms have enzymes and metabolites that function at extreme temperatures, pressures, and environments that make them extremely valuable for industry.

There are minor salivary glands on the surface of the tongue that encircle taste buds and produce lingual lipase.

The Fart Side: Blowing in the Wind!

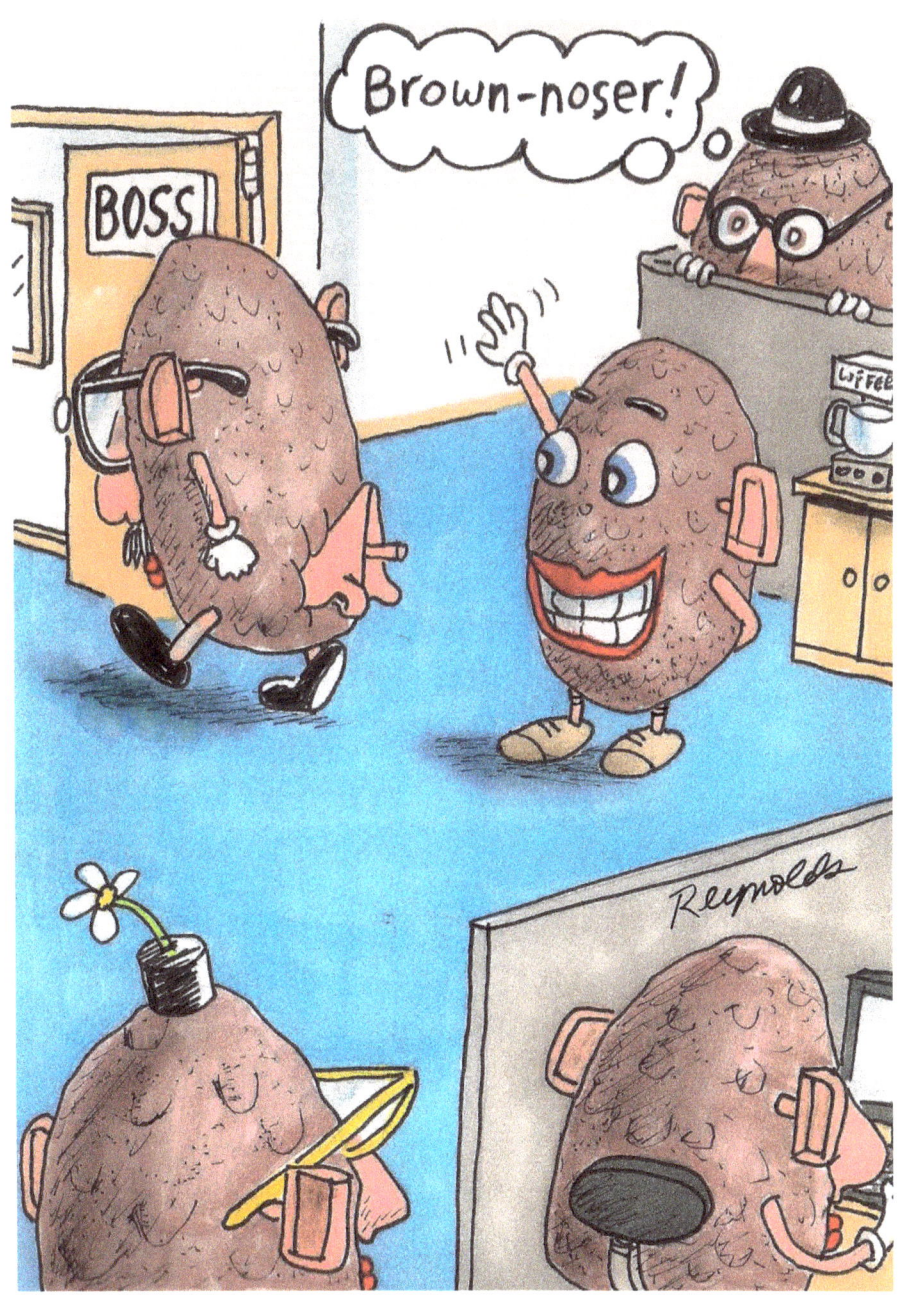

Mad Cow Disease is an infectious disease caused by prions, an entirely new life form recently discovered that does not contain DNA.

Twenty-five percent of the world methane production, which contributes to global warming, comes from termite farts. The gas is produced in their digestive tracts by methanogen Archaea.

When early scientists filtered a liquid free of bacteria, and it still caused disease, they assumed it was a poison secreted by the bacteria. They gave it the Latin name for poison, virus. When it was identified as a separate and new life form, they left the name intact even though it is a misnomer.

The main salivary glands are exocrine glands which secrete saliva via ducts that drain into the mouth.

The Fart Side: Blowing in the Wind!

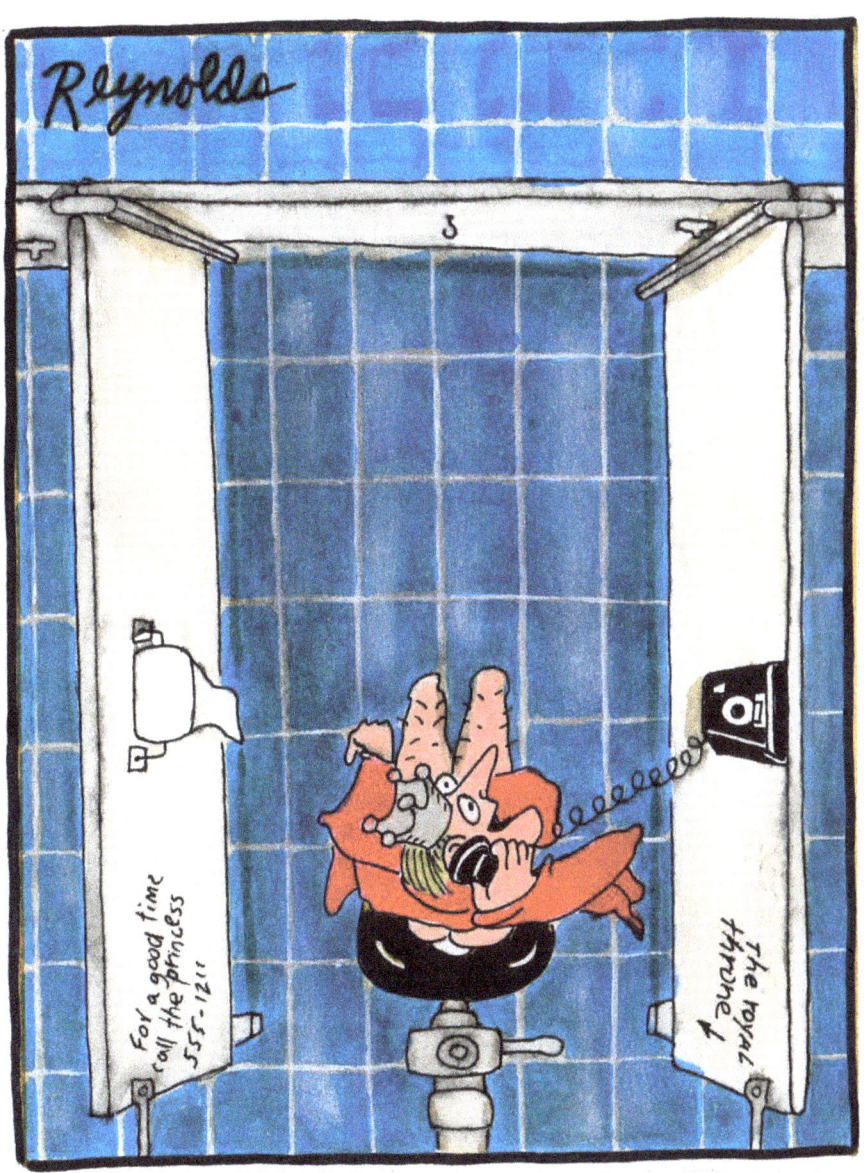

"Why, yes! As a matter-of-fact this is Prince Albert in a can."

In Ancient Rome, military discipline for disloyal soldiers was that every group of ten were to draw lots to identify the one soldier to be murdered by his fellow soldiers. The Latin term used to identify the removal of one tenth was the origin of the word decimation.

The bacteriophage virus can effectively kill bacteria by infecting them. They produce more virus particles inside the bacterial cell in such large numbers that the cell explodes, further spreading the virus. River water containing large numbers of viral bacteriophages have been used to treat bacterial infections over one hundred years ago, before the development of antibiotics.

There are three pairs of main salivary glands, and between 800 and 1,000 minor salivary glands.

The Fart Side: Blowing in the Wind!

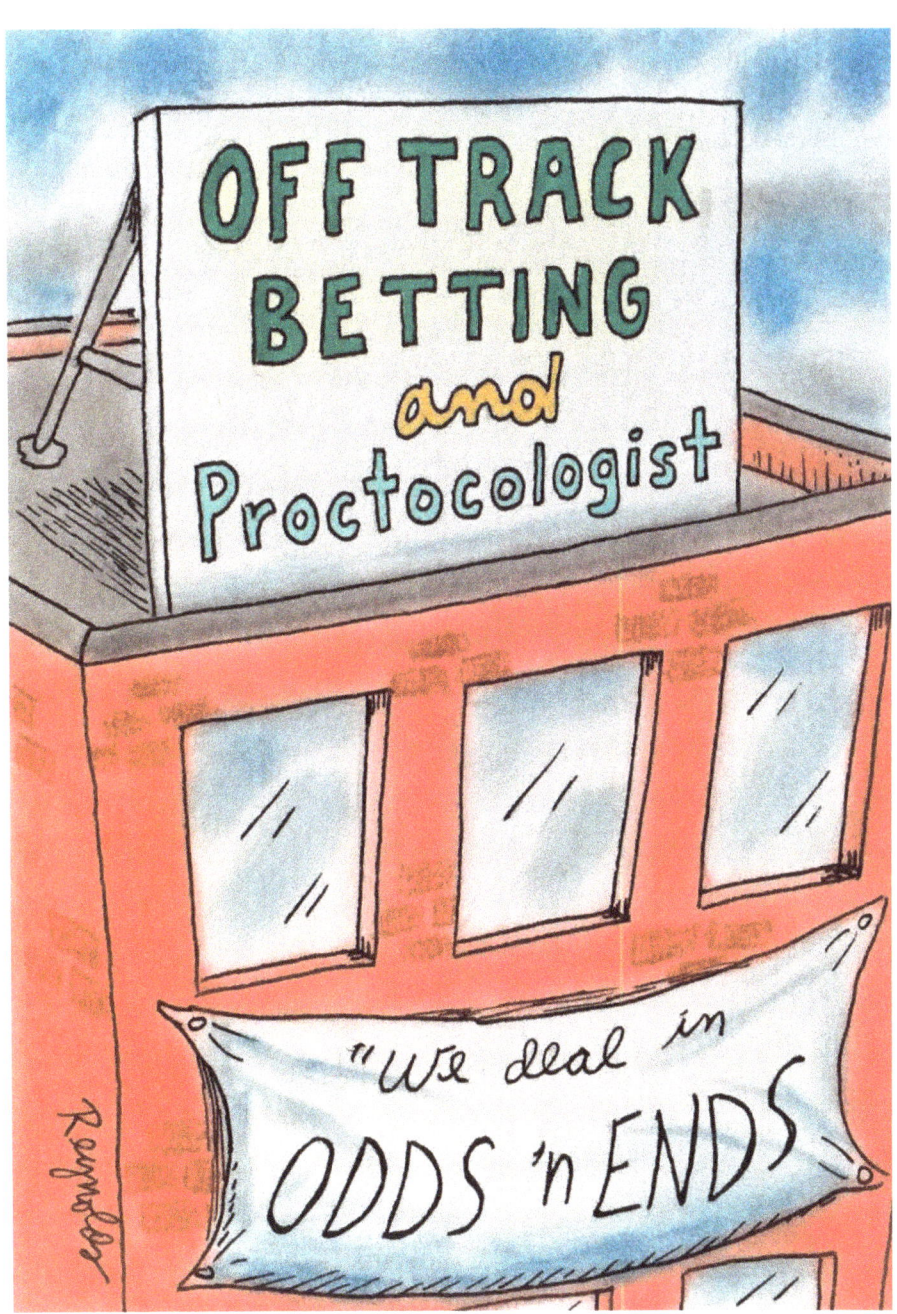

It is estimated that seventy percent of the native population of the Americas perished because they did not have immunity to the communicable diseases brought by the colonists.

Termites trapped in amber, the thousands of years old petrified sap of trees, have preserved pockets of fart gas that still contain the methane that the termites passed. The methane was produced by the Archaea organisms in the termite guts which fermented the cellulose in their diet.

The large intestine is approximately five feet long (one and one-half meters).

The cellular organelles mitochondria and chloroplasts are thought to have been previously independent organisms that were subsequently incorporated into the cells.

The Fart Side: Blowing in the Wind!

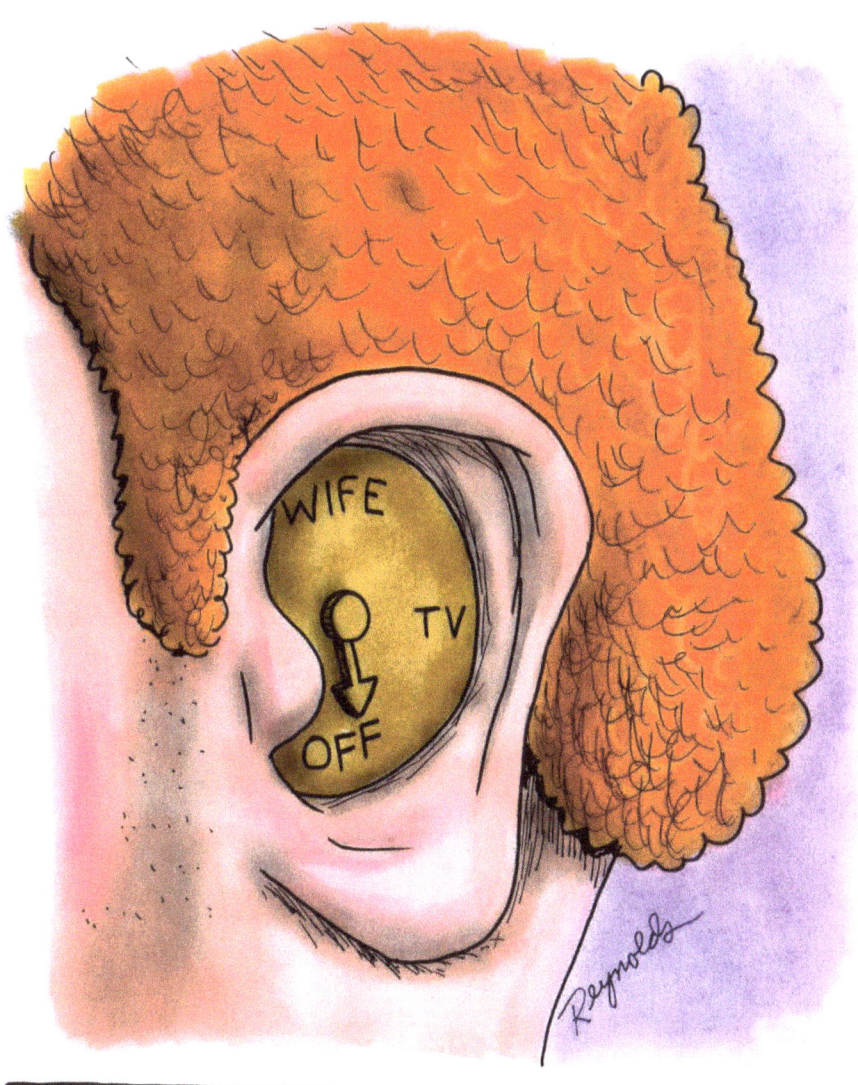

The ability of many organisms such as Archaea to survive extreme conditions adds validity to the theory that life may have come to Earth from other planets, or preexist elsewhere in the universe, a field described as astrobiology.

Human bite injuries are considered more dangerous than dog and animal bites.

Pregnant woman should never change a kitty litter box, and are advised to stay away from cats, because of the risk of acquiring the common parasite *Toxoplasma gondii*. It can lead to fetal involvement and complications.

The giant lizard known as the Komodo Dragon can kill with its bite, but often it is only because the virulent bacteria in its mouth cause deadly infections.

The Fart Side: Blowing in the Wind!

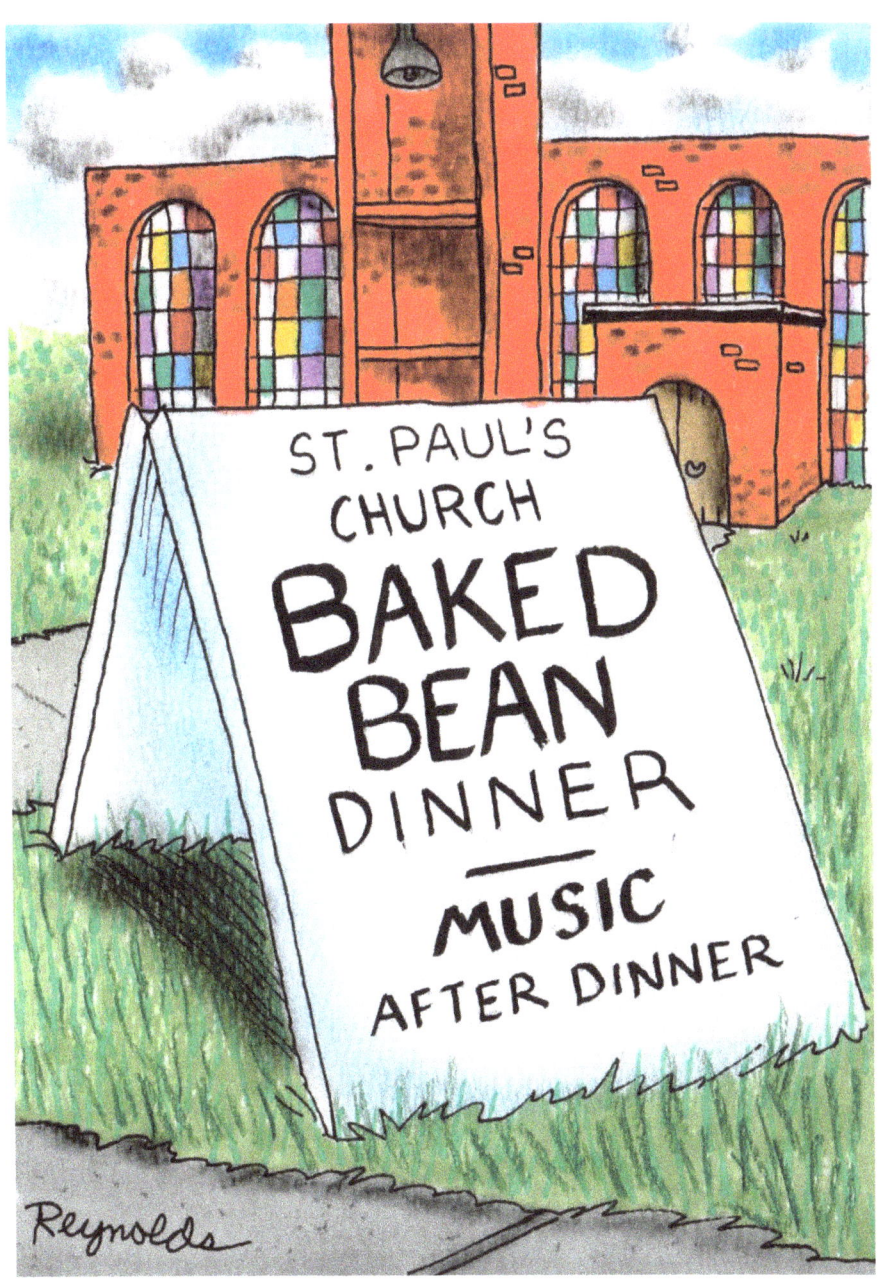

The sea cucumber, if threatened, will discard its digestive tract which continues to move and acts as a decoy as the organism escapes to survive and grow another.

Women produce more of the hydrogen sulfide gas which has a foul rotten egg smell than men.

Humans produce on average one to two liters (quarts) of saliva per day.

The medical term for swallowing is deglutition.

Indole is a compound that contributes to the characteristic smell of feces. At low concentrations, it has a flowery aroma and is used in perfumes.

Thirty percent of fat is hydrolyzed in by the lingual lipase alone within a period of one to twenty minutes.

The Fart Side: Blowing in the Wind!

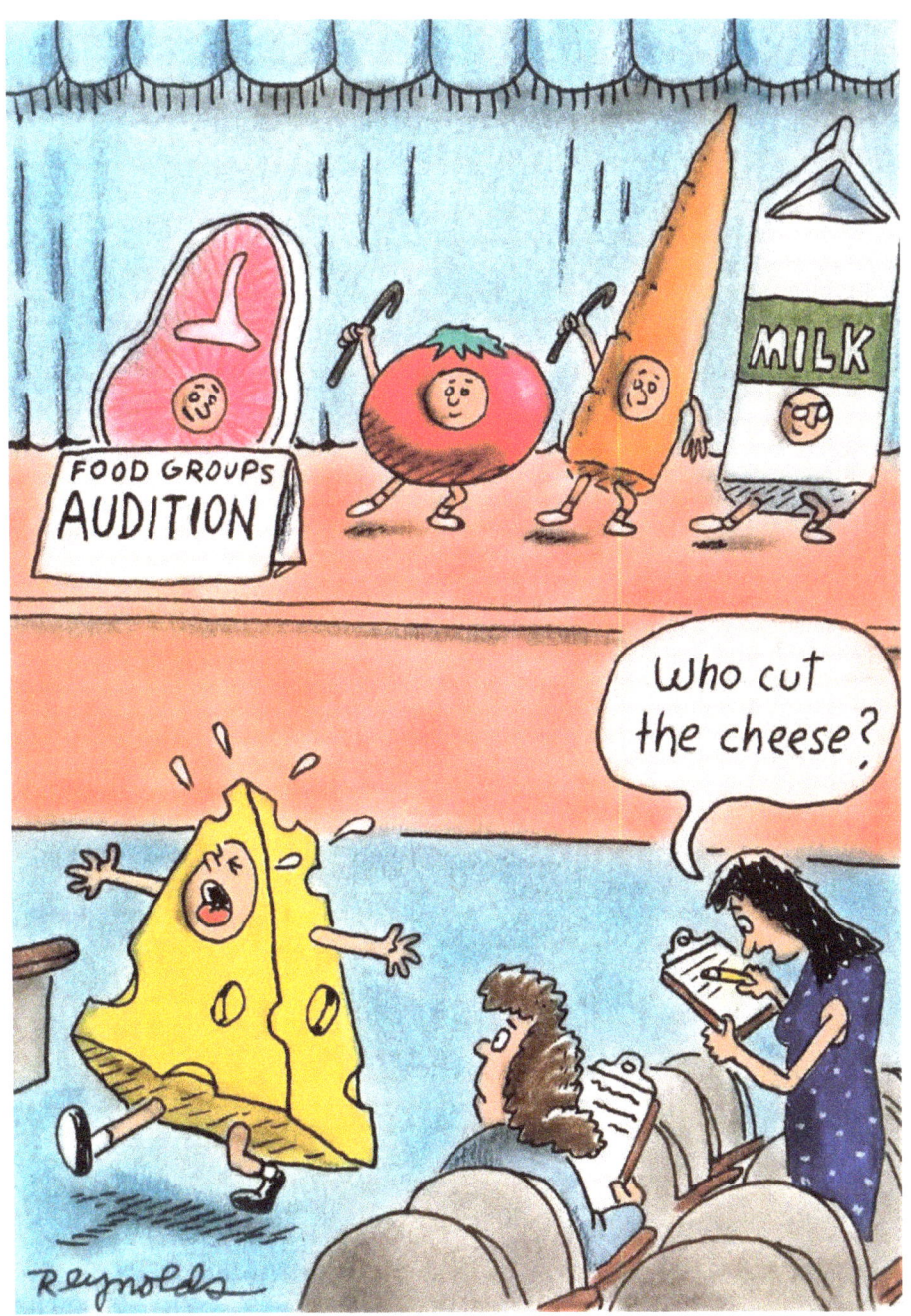

The Chinese delicacy of bird nest soup is made from the saliva of birds.

Snake saliva is its poisonous venom, which can be delivered by fangs or by spitting, often at a distance of up to eight feet.

Simethicone works by decreasing surface tension to make large bubbles smaller.

Yoga breathing techniques stimulate the vagus nerve and may have significant health benefits.

Electrical stimulation of the vagus nerve is an FDA approved treatment for depression.

Every ten years, adults rebuild and remodel every bone in the body. The body needs calcium, magnesium, boron and Vitamin D to do so.

The Fart Side: Blowing in the Wind!

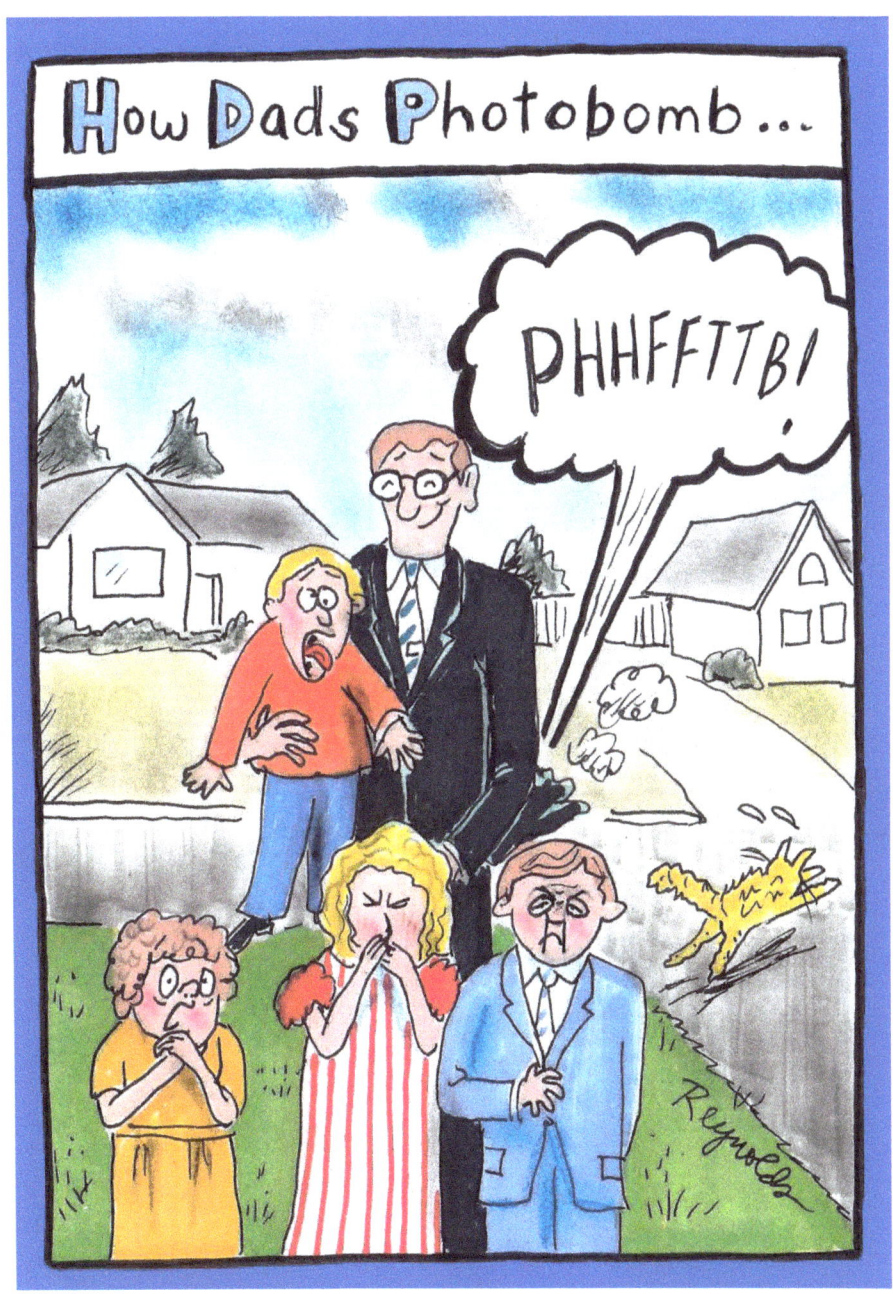

Elagabalus, a Roman Emperor who was assassinated at age eighteen, was known for using whoopee cushions as a practical joke.

Fructose is twice as sweet as the table sugar sucrose.

The average person spends a range from six months to three years of their life sitting on the toilet.

Birds will swallow small stones on purpose to be used in their gizzard to aid in digestion.

The growth of disease causing (pathogenic) bacteria in your gut is controlled by the presence of populations of beneficial bacteria which compete with them for nutrition.

Methane in a fart is odorless

The Fart Side: Blowing in the Wind!

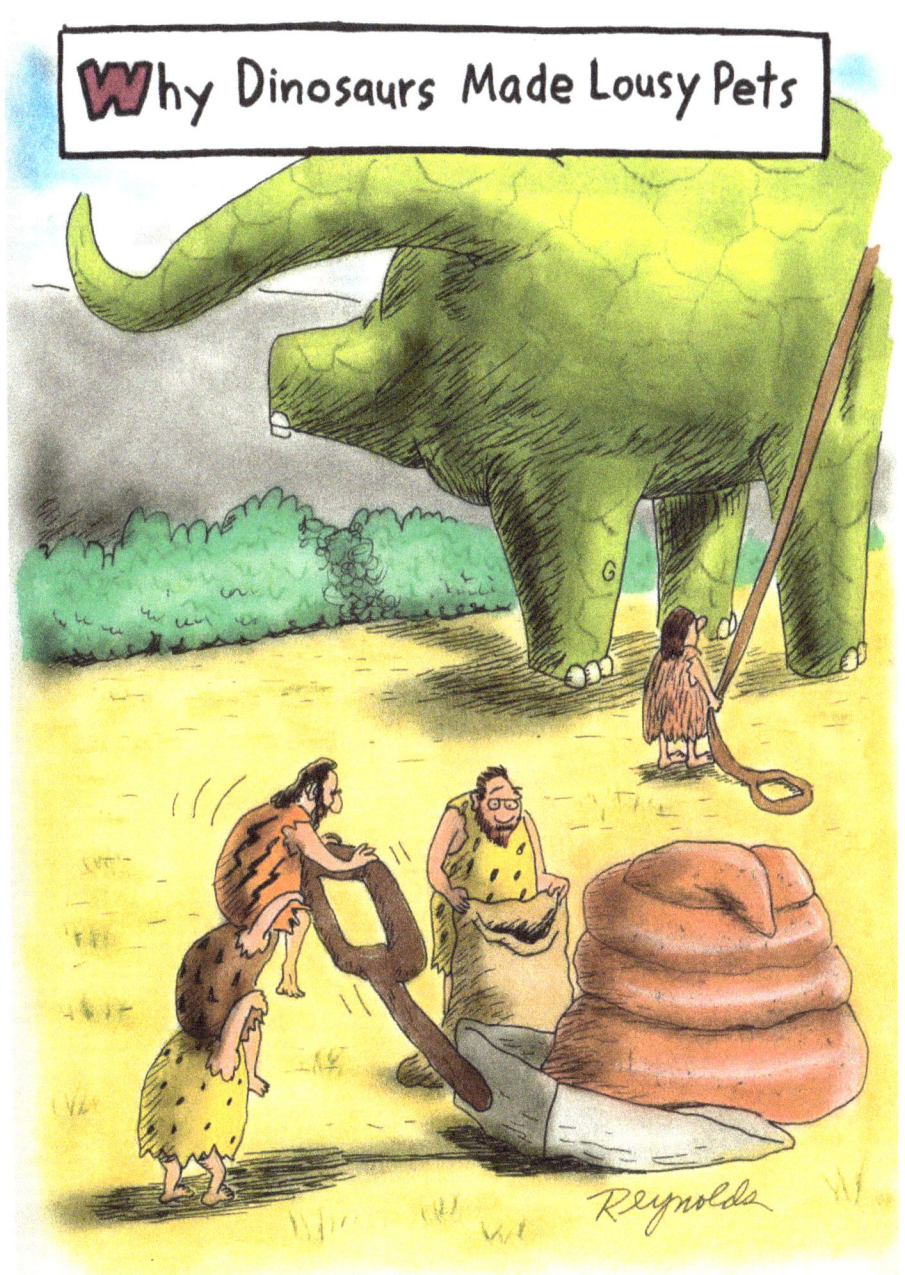

One third of Americans flush the toilet while still sitting on it.

Not all life forms have cells that contain a nucleus.

A glass can be filled with water that goes over the brim without spilling. The physical principle that explains this phenomenon is known as surface tension

There are over six thousand different languages in use humans.

Humans and primitive microbes share thousands of identical genes.

The human genome is less complex than the genomes of many fruits and vegetables.

Vitamin D is mislabeled as a vitamin. It is actually a hormone.

The Fart Side: Blowing in the Wind!

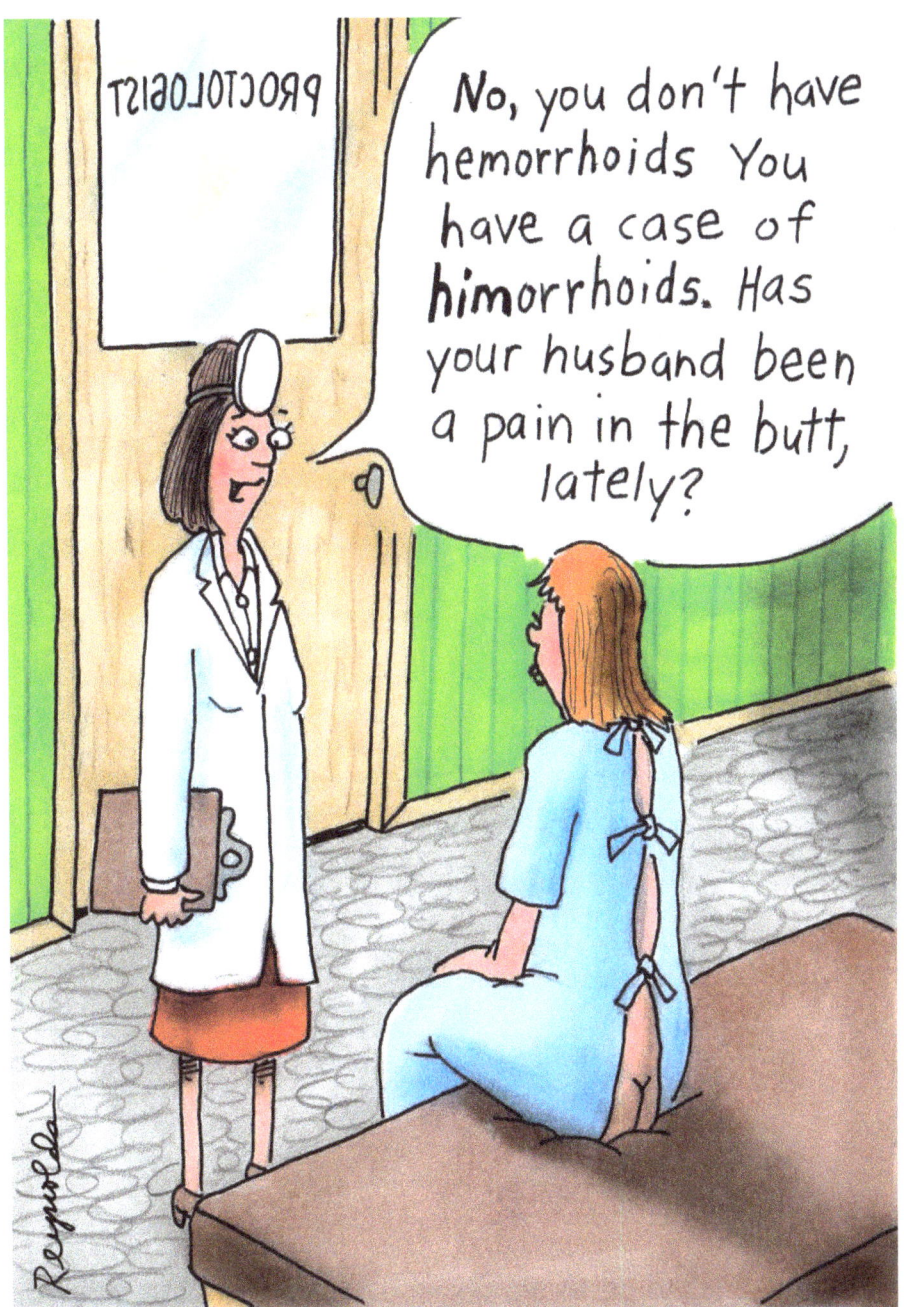

Ronald Wilson Reagan (1911 – 2004) was the fortieth President of the United Sates. An apocryphal story is related to Her Majesty, Queen Elizabeth II of Great Britain who was visiting the presidential ranch, Rancho Cielo, in the Santa Ynez Mountains of California.

The ranch is at a high elevation (Rancho Cielo is Spanish for Sky Ranch) and as both the president and queen are horse aficionados they went for a ride on the ranch trails. At higher altitude, the atmospheric pressure is less than at sea level and thus the volume of gasses expands (Boyle's Law).

The horse's intestinal tract likewise experienced expanding gasses, and being natural animals they release it at will, even if they are in the presence of a Royal Queen and President. Along

the trail the Queen's horse became increasingly flatulent, with noisy and pungent emissions.

The smell became overwhelming and unbearable, and the Queen felt obliged to apologize for her horse's gassiness by making the following comment to Mr. Reagan:

"Mr. President, I really must apologize for the terrible aroma."

Mr. Reagan politely responded, "Your Majesty, you needn't have apologized at all. In fact, if you hadn't said anything, I would have thought it was the horses!

The Funny Side Collection

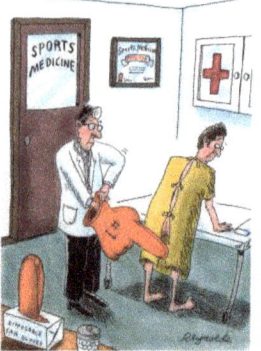

Dan Reynolds
Joseph Weiss, MD

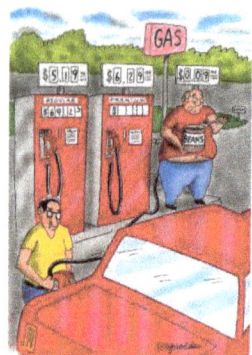

Dan Reynolds
Joseph Weiss, MD

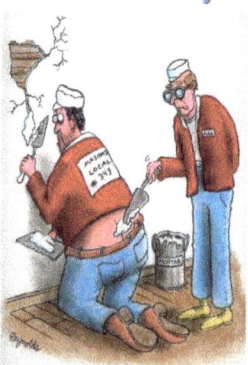

Dan Reynolds
Joseph Weiss, MD

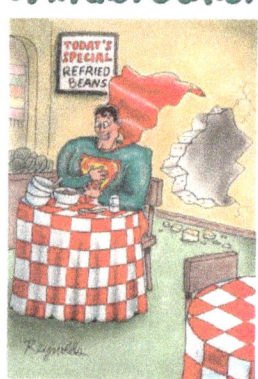

Dan Reynolds
Joseph Weiss, MD

Available in 5"x7" (96 pages) Pocket Rocket! & 6"x9" (122 pages) Expanded Full Blast! print/e-book edition

www.thefunnysidecollection.com

The Fart Side: Blowing in the Wind!

Dan Reynolds

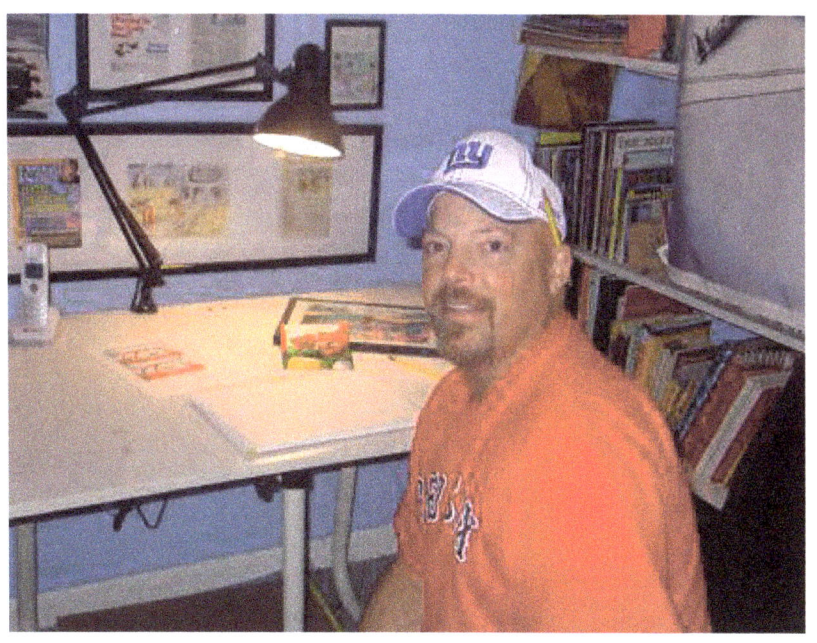

Dan Reynolds began drawing cartoons in December of 1989. He draws and eats left-handed. He plays ping pong and pool left-handed. He throws, kicks and bats right-handed. Like a box of chocolates, you never know what you're going to get, but you will like most of them and they'll keep you coming back. Unlike chocolates, REYNOLDS UNWRAPPED cartoons are not fattening.

The Funny Side Collection

Dan's cartoons are seen by millions of readers across the U.S., Canada, and points beyond all the way down under in Australia. His work is seen in every issue of Reader's Digest (where he is known for his cow, pig and chicken cartoons).

His cartoons have appeared on HBO's The Sopranos, the cover of a National Lampoon cartoon book collection, and on greeting cards all throughout the United States. His work also appears in many other places as well.

Sign-up for Dan's daily REYNOLDS UNWRAPPED e-mail cartoon for only $12 for a whole year. E-mail Dan at reynoldsunwrapped@gmail.com for details. Dan's website is: **www.reynoldsunwrapped.weebly.com**

The Fart Side series and other items are available at:
www.thefunnysidecollection.com

The Fart Side: Blowing in the Wind!

Joseph Weiss, M.D.

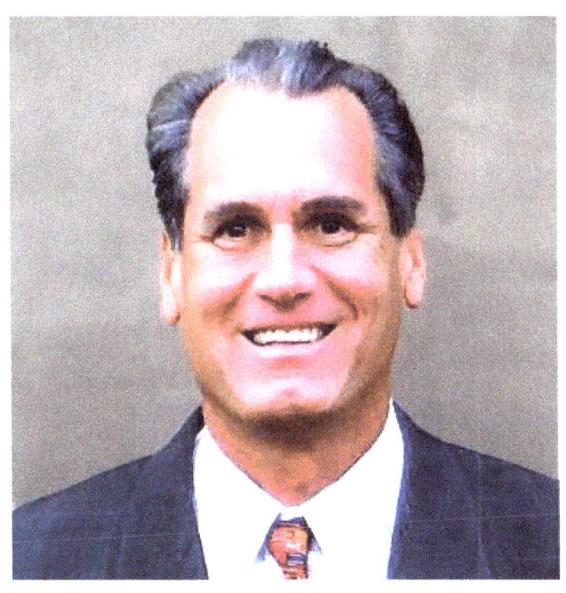

GI Joe is Clinical Professor of Medicine in the Division of Gastroenterology at the University of California, San Diego. He is a Fellow of the American College of Physicians, Fellow of the American Gastroenterological Association, and a Senior Fellow of the American College of Gastroenterology.

Dr. Weiss is the author of several dozen books on health available at:
www.smartaskbooks.com

The Funny Side Collection

He is an accomplished professional speaker and humorist, having given over three thousand invited presentations internationally at universities, international conventions, conferences, corporations, resorts, and special events.

The Fart Side series and other items are available at:
www.thefunnysidecollection.com

"Dr. Joseph Weiss' books provide an informative and entertaining approach to sharing insights about our digestive system and wellbeing." **Deepak Chopra, MD**

"Joseph Weiss, M.D. has a gift for books that are uniquely informative and entertaining. **Jack Canfield** Coauthor of the Chicken Soup for the Soul® series

The Fart Side: Blowing in the Wind!

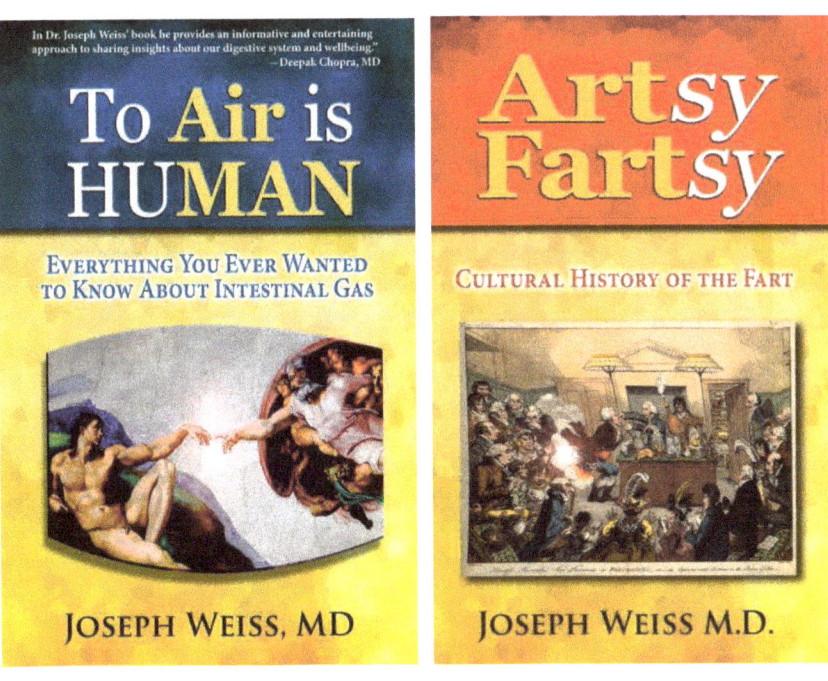

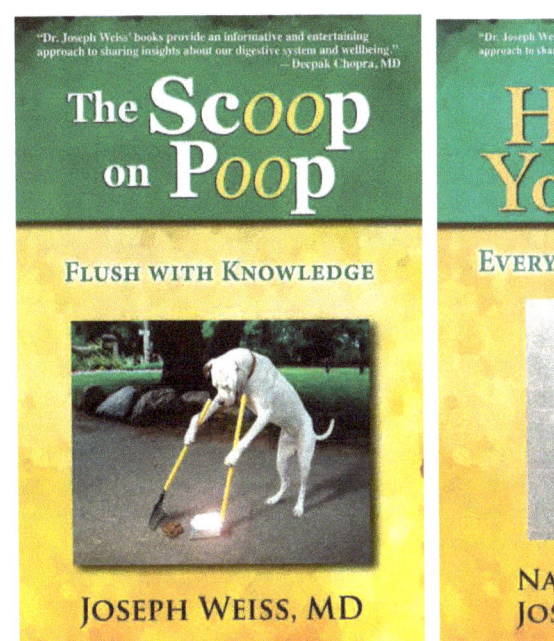

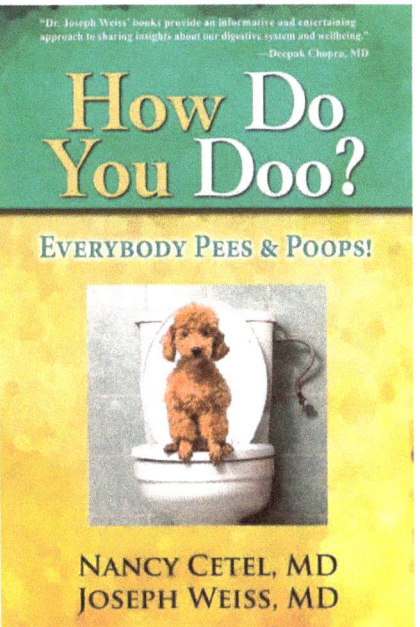

www.smartaskbooks.com

The Funny Side Collection

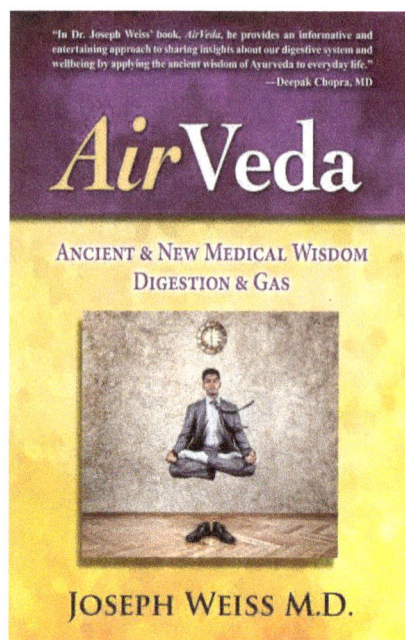
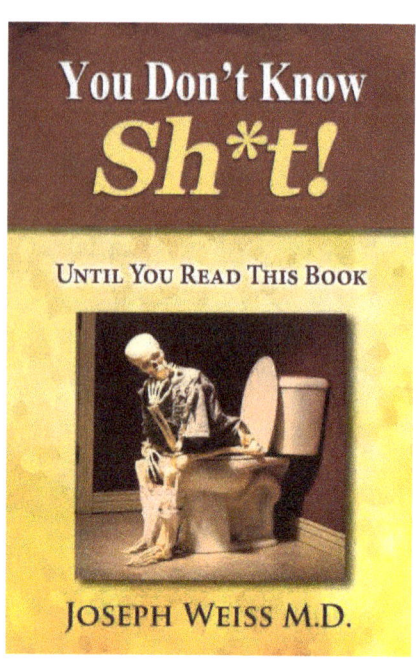
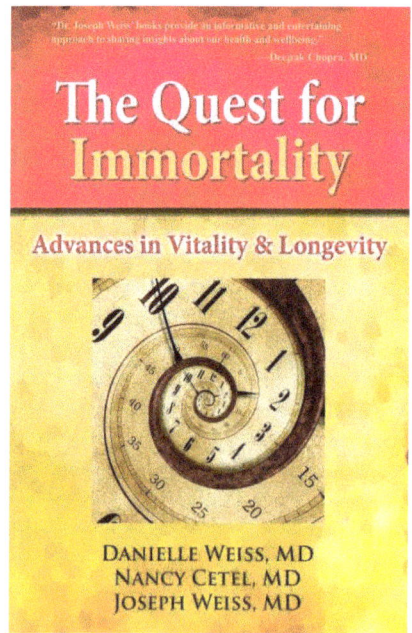
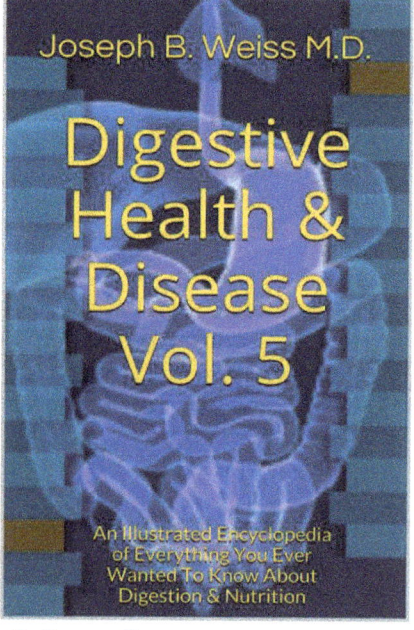

www.smartaskbooks.com

www.ingramcontent.com/pod-product-compliance
Lightning Source LLC
Chambersburg PA
CBHW041958080526
44588CB00021B/2784